DATE DUE

APR 2 2 2001			
GAYLORD			PRINTED IN U.S.A.

ENGINEERING THEORY IN ORTHOPAEDICS:
An Introduction

ENGINEERING THEORY IN ORTHOPAEDICS:
An Introduction

Editors:

M. GREEN and L. D. M. NOKES
Fracture Dynamics and Healing Research Group
Department of Mechanical and Manufacturing Systems Engineering
University of Wales Institute of Science and Technology, Cardiff

ELLIS HORWOOD LIMITED
Publishers · Chichester

Halsted Press: a division of
JOHN WILEY & SONS
New York · Chichester · Brisbane · Toronto

First published in 1988 by
ELLIS HORWOOD LIMITED
Market Cross House, Cooper Street,
Chichester, West Sussex, PO19 1EB, England
The publisher's colophon is reproduced from James Gillison's drawing of the ancient Market Cross, Chichester.

Distributors:

Australia and New Zealand:
JACARANDA WILEY LIMITED
GPO Box 859, Brisbane, Queensland 4001, Australia

Canada:
JOHN WILEY & SONS CANADA LIMITED
22 Worcester Road, Rexdale, Ontario, Canada

Europe and Africa:
JOHN WILEY & SONS LIMITED
Baffins Lane, Chichester, West Sussex, England

North and South America and the rest of the world:
Halsted Press: a division of
JOHN WILEY & SONS
605 Third Avenue, New York, NY 10158, USA

South-East Asia
JOHN WILEY & SONS (SEA) PTE LIMITED
37 Jalan Pemimpin # 05–04
Block B, Union Industrial Building, Singapore 2057

Indian Subcontinent
WILEY EASTERN LIMITED
4835/24 Ansari Road
Daryaganj, New Delhi 110002, India

British Library Cataloguing in Publication Data
Engineering theory in orthopaedics.
1. Medicine. Orthopaedics. Applications of biomechanics.
I. Green, M. (Michael), *1960–* II. Nokes, L. D. M.
6.17'3
Library of Congress CIP available

ISBN 0–7458–0337–7 (Ellis Horwood Limited)
ISBN 0–470–21261–6 (Halsted Press)

Typeset in Times by Ellis Horwood Limited
Printed in Great Britain by Hartnolls, Bodmin

The authors

H. CLARKE
Lecturer in Materials, Department of Mechanical and Manufacturing Systems Engineering, University of Wales Institute of Science and Technology, PO Box 25, Cardiff, CF1 3XE, UK

Dr M. GREEN
University of Wales Research Fellow, Department of Mechanical and Manufacturing Systems Engineering, University of Wales Institute of Science and Technology, PO Box 25, Cardiff, CF1 3XE, UK

I. G. MACKIE, FRCS
Senior Lecturer in Orthopaedics, Department of Traumatic and Orthopaedic Surgery, University of Wales College of Medicine, Cardiff, UK

W. J. MINTOWT-CZYZ, FRCS
Consultant in Orthopaedic Surgery, Royal Gwent Hospital, Newport, Gwent, UK

Dr L. D. M. NOKES
Lecturer,Department of Mechanical and Manufacturing Systems Engineering, University of Wales Institute of Science and Technology, PO Box 25, Cardiff, CF1 3XE, UK

Dr J. RICHARDS
Lecturer in Engineering, Department of Mechanical and Manufacturing Systems Engineering, University of Wales Institute of Science and Technology, PO Box 25, Cardiff, CF1 3XE, UK

Table of contents

Foreword

The advance made during the past few decades in the field of medicine have been truly remarkable. Such advances, however, can only be achieved from the solid base provided by a firm grasp of the underlying principles which are fundamental to the field of study. Thus, in recent years, as the pace of advancement has increased, the advantages of a multidisciplinary approach to research and development have come to the fore. It is with this in mind that I welcome this book and the course on which it is based.

Having been involved in the design and production of prostheses and implants for many years, I know from experience that both engineers and surgeons must have an understanding of the problems faced on a daily basis by the other. A cross-fertilization of ideas between the engineers who design and produce implants and the surgeons who ultimately use them is therefore vital and must be encouraged if we are to achieve the aim of all engaged in this work, that is to provide the best possible treatment for the people who matter the most — the patients.

It is with this backdrop of experience that, with great honour, I am pleased to write this foreword to an excellent contribution to bioengineering.

Dane A. Miller, PhD
President
Biomet Inc.

Preface

The recent trend towards a multidisciplinary approach to Biomechanical Engineering is to be applauded. In this volume, we have attempted to outline the basics of engineering and materials theory applicable to orthopaedic surgery. It is our hope that this volume will inspire further study and research in this field which will ultimately be to the benefit of the people who matter most — the patients.

We are greatly indebted to our co-authors for their contributions and to Mrs C. Merridew and Mr D. Thomas for their aid in the production of this work.

Any errors and omissions, of course, remain our responsibility.

Cardiff, 1988   M. Green,
                                                                L. D. M. Nokes

1

Materials

H. Clarke and M. Green

INTRODUCTION

The aim of this work is to provide an insight into the basis of engineering theory as applicable to orthopaedic surgery. We have attempted to present the material in such a manner so as to be easily understood by practitioners of both disciplines. This has necessitated, in parts, a simplistic view of some very complex matters, therefore, where appropriate, additional reading lists have been provided.

The limiting factor in many engineering and surgical problems are the mechanical and other properties of the materials available for use in the task at hand. This, therefore, provides us with a useful starting point. First we shall consider the broad field of materials.

PROPERTIES OF MATERIALS

To be able to choose appropriate materials and produce a satisfactory design it is essential to measure the relevant properties of materials. Properties can be broadly classified as physical and mechanical. Physical properties are density, electrical conductivity, resistivity, etc. Mechanical properties of a material describe the behaviour of a material when subject to a force. Absolute values of some properties are hard to determine and are often quoted in comparison with other materials. Mechanical properties may be determined to provide engineering design data or as a quality assessment in the standard for raw materials or manufacturing operations carried out on the material.

Engineers use such terms as strength, brittleness, hardness, when describing material properties and a list of the common terms is given below.

Strength   The ability of a material to resist an applied force without rupture.

Hardness   Usually defined as resistance to indentation although in a number of instances the resistance to wear is important.

Elasticity   The ability of a material to recover its original shape after deformation.

Plasticity   The ability of a material to be formed to a new shape without fracture and retain that shape after load removal.

Ductility   The ability of a material to be stretched without fracture.

Malleability The ability of a material to be compressed into a new shape without fracture.

Toughness   The ability of a material to withstand suddenly applied forces without fracture.

Brittleness   Opposite of toughness; usually there is no evidence of plasticity prior to fracture.

Materials testing

A number of different tests are used to characterize the behaviour of a material under stress. The capacity of a material to withstand static loads can be determined by testing that material in tension or compression. Hardness is measured by assessing resistance to indentation. Impact tests are used to indicate toughness of a material under shock loading. Fatigue tests measure material response to cyclic loading. Creep and stress rupture tests are conducted to evaluate behaviour when the material is subject to load at elevated temperature. The results of such tests are usually of more empirical than fundamental significance. None the less, they are useful to designer and fabricator.

Tensile testing

Of all the tests used to evaluate mechanical properties of materials, this is probably the most useful. To test a material a test piece is first manufactured. The size and shape of these varies appreciably but have a common geometry of form in that they all possess a central parallel section, the gauge length, on which all measurements are made. The ends of the specimen are deliberately larger than this section to ensure that the action of gripping the specimen to apply a force does not affect the result and ensure failure within gauge length. The more important dimensions are:

(1) the gauge length L_0,
(2) initial cross-section area, a_0.

Forces are applied to the test piece via its ends and the effect of such forces measured by recording the extension of a known length on the parallel section. Forces are applied by means of mechanical or hydraulic devices and extension measured by sensitive measuring devices called extensometers. Force is incrementally applied to the specimen and after each increment the extension produced is measured. The force is increased up to the point of failure. Results are usually plotted as force–extension graphs (Fig. 1.1). More mean-

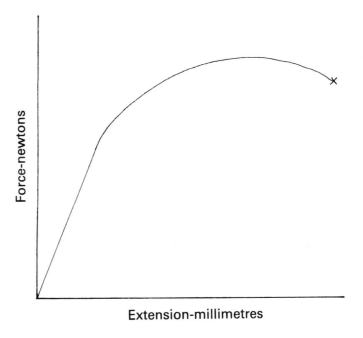

Fig. 1.1 — Typical force–extension relationship.

ingful information can be obtained if a stress–strain graph is plotted. This removes the effect of geometry and allows direct comparison of different materials.

Strain

Strain measures how much a material has stretched under a force. Thus if a rod of length L is stretched by an amount l by the action of a force, the strain, ε, in the material is defined as:

$$\text{Strain} = \frac{\text{increase in length}}{\text{original length}} = \frac{l}{L} = \varepsilon.$$

Units of strain

Since we are dividing one length by another length, strain is a ratio, i.e. a number and has no units. Note that because strains are often numerically quite small, it is common to express then as percentages and reduce possible confusion with decimal points, e.g. $\varepsilon = 0.006$ or 0.6%.

Stress

The stress in a given direction at a point in a material is the force acting on that direction at the point divided by the area on which the force acts.

Units of stress

The basic unit of force is the newton. Usually this is too small a base unit and multiples of this are used, e.g.

kilonewton $\equiv 1000$ newtons
meganewton $\equiv 1$ million newtons or 1×10^6 newtons
giganewton $\equiv 1$ thousand million newtons or 1×10^9 newtons.

Area is expressed as square millimetres (mm^2), square centimetres (cm^2) or square metres (m^2) in the SI system and square inches (in^2) in the traditional unit system.

This leads to the following units of stress:

newtons per square millimetre	$N\ mm^{-2}$
meganewtons per square metre	MN/m^{-2}
pounds (force) per square inch	psi
kilograms (force) per square centimetre	$kg(f)\ cm^{-2}$
$1\ MN\ m^{-2} = 10.2\ kg(f)\ cm^{-2} = 146$ psi	

Stress tells us how hard atoms/molecules in a solid are being pulled apart by external forces.

Strain tells us how far atoms/molecules are being pulled apart.

Stress–strain diagrams
Each force value is divided by the original area of cross-section of the
parallel section of the test pieces and each extension by the original
length. This does not alter the general form of the graph but merely
rescales the axes used. A typical curve is reproduced in Fig. 1.2.

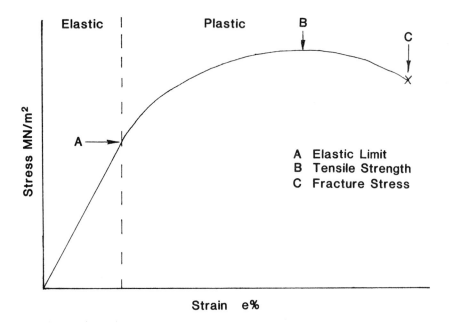

Fig. 1.2 — Typical stress–strain relationship.

At the beginning of the test the material behaves elastically, i.e.
removal of the stress allows the sample to return to its original length.
A material is said to have been plastically deformed if, on removal of
the load, the material does not return to its original length. In the
most general case, the elongation of the test piece comprises two
parts, an elastic part and a plastic part. The elastic part contains both
time dependent and time independent contributions, although for
metals the former is ignored. Fig. 1.2 shows typical elastic behaviour
of real solids.

The plastic part includes a region of uniform elongation in which
all portions of the specimen extend by the same amount and a non-
uniform part in which localized deformation or cracking occurs
(rapidly followed by fracture). Sometimes fracture only occurs in the
elastic region and the material is said to be brittle. The term brittle is

also applied to materials which show limited amounts of plastic deformation prior to fracture. A typical stress–strain diagram showing the various regions is given in Fig. 1.3.

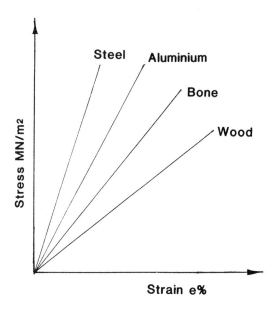

Fig. 1.3 — Typical elastic behaviour of real solids.

For some materials (mild steel) the transition from elastic to plastic behaviour is readily identified by a marked 'kink' in the stress–strain curve, thus it is referred to as the yield point. For the majority of materials the transition is less apparent and can be strain rate sensitive. Where it is difficult to determine the transition, an arbitrary yield point is defined in terms of a proof stress. The proof stress is the stress at which a permanent extension of a specified percentage of the gauge length (usually 0.2%) occurs.

The figure of 0.2% extension gives some indication of the relative proportions of elastic and plastic deformation when it is realized that the strain to fracture can be up to 80% for metals and some 1000% for thermoplastics.

Most components or assemblies of components in engineering are designed to resist excessive deflection and not permanently deform under load and hence it is the elastic region of the curve which is of interest and it is usual to limit the allowable stress in a component to some fraction of yield or proof stress, i.e. a factor of safety is employed.

When considering how a material will behave during manufacture, it is the plastic component of the strain which is important; the greater the strain to failure the greater the capacity of the material to be forced into a new configuration without breaking.

A number of properties which can be used to characterize the material are derived from the tensile test. These are as follows.

Elastic modulus

For the elastic region of the stress–strain curve, the ratio of stress (σ) to strain (ε) is constant. This constant is termed Young's modulus of elasticity and is designated by the symbol E. The modulus is a measure of the stiffness of a material and the higher its value, i.e. the steeper the slope of the σ–ε curve, the stiffer the material. Ceramics tend to show the highest values. Metals and polymers exhibit a wide range of values. However, it should be noted, for reasons to be explained later, that the values ascribed to polymers are dependent on the strain rate used to determine them. With the exception of some polymers, structural materials show little alteration in stiffness when alloying adjustments are made.

Poisson's ratio

If a piece of rubber is stretched it gets noticeably thinner and conversely if it is compressed it will bulge out sideways. Similar effects occur in materials like steel and bone but the longitudinal and lateral strains are too small to be discernible with the eye. The effect was first observed by Poisson who discovered that the ratio of the lateral strain (e_2) to longitudinal strain (e_1) was constant for a given material. The ratio e_2/e_1 has become known as Poisson's ratio. For most materials its value lies between a quarter and a half. For biological soft tissue the value is about half and for membranes the figure is approximately one.

Yield stress/proof stress

This marks the departure from linearity of stress–strain curves. Its significance has been mentioned earlier. Ceramics have the highest values and polymers the lowest.

Tensile strength

This is the maximum value of stress recorded on the stress–strain curve. No great significance should be attached to this parameter since the true stress (load/current area of cross-section) at this strain value is much larger. Nevertheless, it is a commonly quoted parameter in material specification.

Percentage elongation (to fracture)
This is the permanent elongation of the gauge length after fracture, expressed as a percentage of the original gauge length. If L_F is gauge length after fracture and L_0 the initial gauge length, then:

$$\% \text{ elongation} = \left(\frac{L_F - L_0}{L_0}\right) \times 100$$

This parameter may be regarded as the measure of the plasticity of a material, i.e. its ductility. Useful ductile materials show values as high as 80%. The main use of the parameter is in predicting possible behaviour during cold deformation processes, e.g. bending to shape. The higher the percentage elongation, the greater the amount of deformation that can be carried out on a material before fracture begins. For metals it may also be used to give an indication of how much coldwork may be used to raise the yield stress of the material without risking fracture. It is difficult to link this parameter directly with any design requirement because the stresses applied to engineering components/structure parts are deliberately kept below the yield stress where plastic strain is absent. However, engineers still like to use ductile materials to manufacture components. The reasons for this are probably twofold.

(a) The amount of plastic yielding gives an indication of overstrain and is an added safety feature.
(b) The existence of ductility helps to guard against the serious consequences of stress concentrations (about which more will be said in a later section).

A minimum value of 5% is usually required for these purposes. The lack of ductility is a major reason why ceramics as yet have limited application.

Percentage reduction in area
This is an alternative measure of ductility and is defined as the percentage decrease in area of cross-section.

Shear testing
In addition to tension and compression, structures may be subject to shear. The simplest example of shear is the behaviour of a pack of cards when thrown onto a table.

Shear stress
This is a measure of the tendency of one part of a solid to slide past the adjacent part. Shear stress is defined as the ratio:

$$\frac{\text{Shear force}}{\text{Area being sheared}} = \frac{P}{A}$$

The units are the same as those for tensile stress.

Shear strain
A solid will be deformed under the action of a shear stress. However, the deformation (strain) is measured as an angle and is measured in radians. Radians have no dimensions being a ratio. The symbol ϕ is used for angular strain (Fig. 1.4).

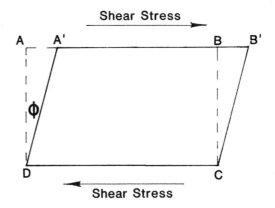

Shear Strain $=\underline{/ADA'} \simeq \dfrac{AA'}{AD}$ rad

Fig. 1.4 — Measurement of shear stress.

Shear modulus
Materials subject to shear stress obey Hooke's law in the elastic range and a shear stress–shear strain curve will be very similar to a tensile stress–strain curve. The gradient of the straight part of the curve

represents the stiffness of a material in shear and is called the shear modulus, G.

$$G = \frac{\text{Shear stress}}{\text{Shear strain}}$$

G has dimensions and units of stress, e.g. MN m^{-2}.

Time-dependent mechanical properties
The simple tensile tests discussed above are performed in a matter of minutes. Such tests do not identify those materials (e.g. polymers) which are strain rate sensitive. For metals application of a stress, below the yield stress, at ambient temperatures, produces a strain which will not alter in value with time. Thermoplastic polymers on the other hand will show a progressive increase of strain with time. A typical variation of strain with time is illustrated in Fig. 1.5 This

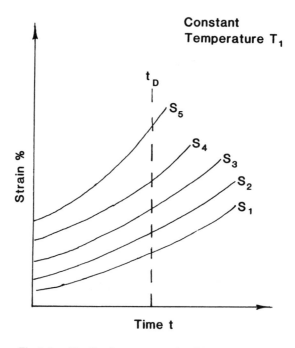

Fig. 1.5 — Family of creep curves for different stresses S_x.

means, of course, that the modulus of elasticity will be a function of time.

If either stress or temperature are altered the form of the curve alters and it is normal to provide information on the effect of stress or temperature variation. A typical representation is given in Fig. 1.5, where increasing constant stress levels are used to establish families of creep curves.

This dependence on time, stress level and temperature makes it difficult to establish usable data for design purposes. A number of techniques have evolved to deal with the problem; one of these being the construction of isochronous curves. The construction is illustrated in Figs 1.5 and 1.6.

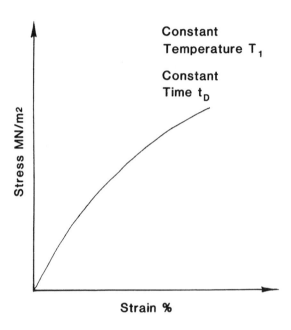

Fig. 1.6 — Isochronous curve derived from creep data.

A design time, τ_D, is identified for the application. The strains corresponding to this loading time are established for each stress level (Fig. 1.5). A curve relating stress to strain is drawn for this loading time (Fig. 1.6). This relationship may not be linear. The slope of the isochronous stress–strain curve gives a modulus value, E_{τ_D}. This time-dependent modulus value may be used in standard engineering design formulae.

The effects of temperature may be assessed by determining isochronous curves at different temperatures.

Compression testing

These are rarely carried out on ductile metals because surface friction at the loading points constrain the sample. However, the test is commonly used for brittle materials which, because of their sensitivity to surface cracks, produce large variations in strength. The test establishes yield and compression strengths in a similar manner to tensile tests.

Fatigue testing

It is now well established that a material cannot withstand as high a stress under long periods of cycle loading as it can under static loading. Yield strength and tensile strength are useful measures of load carrying ability under static loading only. A fatigue test determines the number of cycles of stress a material can withstand. The simplest form of fatigue test is that employing reverse bending where the stress varies between fixed values of tension and compression and the mean stress is zero.

One end of the test piece is held in a rotating clamp and the other loaded via a ball-bearing race (Fig. 1.7). With each rotation all points

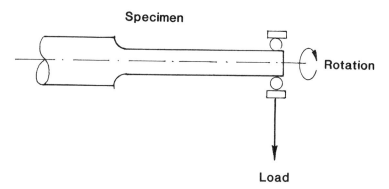

Fig. 1.7 — Fatigue testing in rotating bend.

on the circumference pass from a state of tension to one of compression. The reversal occurs several thousand times per minute. The number of cycles of reversed stress to produce failure is recorded for a range of stress levels. The data is then plotted as stress (S) versus the logarithm of the number of cycles to failure (N). Typical curves obtained are in Fig. 1.8.

Note that for ferrous materials, there exists a stress level, termed the fatigue limit, below which failure will not occur.

A large number of factors influence fatigue life and the usual S–N curves show great scatter. The most significant factors affecting

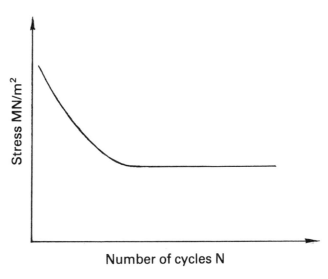

Fig. 1.8 — Typical fatigue curve showing variation of life with stress range.

fatigue life are surface finish and stress concentration — this being related to the fact that most fatigue cracks begin at the surface. Processes, such as shot peening, which produce residual compressive stresses, are employed to reduce their effect. Corrosive environments substantially reduce fatigue life.

Hardness testing
This is used to describe two different, though related, properties, namely resistance to abrasion and resistance to indentation. Resistance to abrasion is assessed by the Mohs' scale of hardness where materials are compared one against another in their ability to scratch each other. More commonly hardness is assessed by indentation tests such as Brinell, Rockwell and Vickers. The most accurate of these is the Vickers test in which a specially shaped diamond is impressed into the surface of a material using a constant load. Hardness is expressed as the ratio load to area of impression made (kg/mm^2). High values indicate hard materials and vice versa.

The test is often used as a cheap substituted for tensile testing since an empirical relationship exists between hardness and tensile strength.

Toughness testing
This could be regarded as the single most important property of a structural material. It is a measure of the energy needed to produce fracture. One assessment of toughness may be obtained by determin-

ing the area under the stress–strain curve. A more empirical
approach has been to use impact tests where the energy to break
standard specimens is determined under rapid loading. A more
modern approach is to use the concept of work of fracture. To break a
material in tension a crack must spread right across it. To create such
a crack requires energy to rupture the atomic bonds holding the
material together and the source of this energy is the strain energy
stored inside the material when it is stressed. The work of fracture
varies widely. For brittle materials such as glass, 1 joule/m^2 of crack
surface is sufficient to cause failure but for mild steel the figure can
rise to 1 000 000 joules/m^2 of crack surface. Brittle materials are not
brittle because of their tensile strengths but because of the low energy
needed to break them. This is why it is inadequate to design on the
basis of tensile strength. The same property also explains why certain
materials are sensitive to stress concentrations. The modern method
of measuring resistance to fracture is fracture toughness. This
assesses how large a crack can be tolerated in a component if it is not
to fail under an applied stress.

The conventional way of measuring toughness is by using the Izod
or Charpy impact test. Here the energy to fracture a notched sample
is determined by measuring the energy lost by the impact hammer
used to break the sample. Unfortunately, such tests yield little
numerical information that can be directly used in design. At best it
allows a materials engineer to rank materials in order of increasing
toughness. A major attraction of the test is its ability to assess a
material's response to the presence of notches — notch sensitivity —
and for ferrous metals the temperature for the ductile to brittle
transition.

FRICTION AND WEAR

The employment of artificial joint systems in the human body has
focused attention on the need to provide some information on their
possible lifespan and probable failure modes. In particular, information is needed on the performance of the contact surfaces of real
joints. A considerable body of knowledge exists in conventional
engineering on those design aspects which govern the life of components which undergo relative motion. Much of this knowledge is
transferable to the situation existing in artificial joints. Factors of
major importance in the life of components which undergo relative
motion are friction, wear and lubrication.

Friction

If a block of metal is placed on a metallic surface and an attempt is made to slide it across the surface, while keeping it in contact with that surface, a resistance is experienced and a certain minimum force must be applied to move and keep the block in motion. This resistance is termed the frictional force, F. For any two surfaces in contact the ratio:

$$\frac{\text{minimum force to produce motion}}{\text{normal force pressing the surfaces together}} = \frac{P}{N} \text{ (see Fig. 1.9)}$$

is a constant. This constant is termed the coefficient of friction, U,

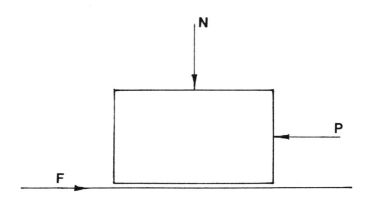

At point of sliding P=F=μN

Fig. 1.9 — Illustration of forces involved in friction.

and its value depends only on the nature of the two surfaces in contact. Typical values of U range from 0.009 in a natural human hip joint to 0.38 for cobalt chrome alloy surfaces in contact. For a given combination of two surfaces the value of the minimum force needed to initiate movement depends only on the normal force which is pressing the two surfaces together; it is not affected by the apparent area of surface in contact.

Frictional forces arise from the interatomic attraction of atoms on opposing surfaces. These atoms are less 'tightly bound' than atoms in the interior. In fact, if the surfaces are perfectly clean, then bringing them into close proximity is sufficient to cause permanent union. Under normal circumstances, the presence of surface contaminants (and a roughened surface) reduces such close contact. Normal machined metal surfaces are seen at high magnification to be very uneven and when such surfaces are placed together the actual area in contact is only a small proportion of the total area. Contact occurs only at local high spots. Application of a force results in extreme localized pressures which flatten such contacts, break up oxide scales and produce solid welding. When an attempt is made to produce relative movement between the two surfaces, these welds have to be broken and this effect is regarded as the source of friction. Increasing the normal load increases the number of cold welds and hence the resistance to sliding.

Lubrication

If a suitable fluid is placed between two surfaces the localized point contacts mentioned above can be reduced or even eliminated. The fluid separates the surfaces and itself undergoes shearing when the two surfaces slide past one another. The fluid also has a resistance to relative motion of the different layers within it; the magnitude of this resistance being related to the viscosity of the fluid. The resistance to shearing in a fluid varies with the rate of shear and can render a lubricant less effective. Fortunately, in the case of the fluid found in human joints, the change of viscosity with shear rate is small and efficient lubrication is obtained even at the low shear rates found in such joints.

Coefficients of friction for the range of materials that have been used in artificial joints have been determined. Values vary with experimental conditions, geometry of surfaces in contact, surface roughness, applied loads, etc. Metal to metal joints show greatest values being some forty times greater than those found in the normal human joints. The nearest approach to the values for the human joint are found to be the PTFE/PTFE combination which is only four times larger. Low friction coefficients are regarded as important in total joint replacement because the frictional force is transmitted to the implant/bone interface and may promote loosening.

Wear

While the friction coefficient is one parameter to consider in the selection of materials for joint replacements, it is widely accepted that the wear resistance of a joint is of far greater importance.

Wear is the name given to the process(es) by which material is removed from one surface by the sliding action of another surface in contact. The material removed may be carried away to another part of the body or it may be repositioned on the surface. A number of wear mechanisms have been identified. These are adhesive wear, abrasive wear, corrosive wear and fatigue wear.

Adhesive wear (also referred to as galling, scuffing or seizing) results from the cold welding action of localized high spots referred to earlier. When cold welded areas rupture, metal is torn from one surface and is left attached to the other. This adhering metal forms a larger projection which can initiate further damage. Metallic debris is also produced. In general, it is the softer metal which suffers damage. Adhesive wear has been identified as the major cause of wear in total joint replacements.

Abrasive wear occurs when a hard surface rubs on a softer one or when hard particles become entrained in the lubricating fluid placed between the surfaces. Material is gouged out from the surface and the resulting debris is not unlike those produced when metals are cut, drilled or turned on a lathe, i.e. small chips or continuous spirals.

Corrosive wear is a combination of corrosion and a wear mechanism. The latter continuously removes protective surface films and permits freshly exposed, reactive metal to dissolve.

Fatigue wear results from a surface being subject to repetitive loading and sliding. The repetitive loading exhausts the ductility of surface layers and eventually produces cracks. Sliding then provides the means to tear material from the lips of the crack and wear ensues.

The wear debris produced by the above mechanisms is distinctive and analysis of such debris can identify the type of wear taking place. Such studies have assisted in the development of suitable material combinations and the establishment of appropriate surface conditions. One aspect of wear in replacement joints is the possible toxic effect of wear debris on human tissue. Work on this aspect is still continuing and may lead to the exclusion of what are otherwise highly wear resistant materials. Current material combinations for hip replacements are the cobalt/chromium alloys and cobalt chrome/high density polyethylene combinations; the latter providing good absorption of shock loads and low friction.

Corrosion

The search for suitable materials to construct artificial joints and implants has been in progress for many years. A perfect implant material is one which is not attacked by the body fluids and has the mechanical properties needed to withstand the imposed loads. Three metals have come into accepted use — stainless steel, cobalt/chromium alloy and titanium — and go a long way to meeting these criteria. However, the desire to use different combinations of metals in implant construction and thus be able to exploit their differing properties has rekindled interest in the behaviour of materials in body fluids. Furthermore, the discovery that even apparently inert non-metallics suffer corrosion and degradation of strength, has reinforced this interest.

Electrochemical corrosion of metals

The manner in which materials degrade in the atmosphere and the mechanisms involved are well documented (see Further Reading). For the particular environment of the human body, only those mechanisms involving electrochemical action need to be studied. The basic corrosion mechanism may be represented by the equation:

$$M_{\text{metal}} \rightarrow M^{n+}_{\text{solution}} + n\,e^{-}_{\text{metal}}$$

where M represents an atom of metal in the solid, M^{n+} the corresponding metal ion produced when n electrons are stripped away. (n is the valency of the metal.) In a closed system a reverse reaction also occurs and eventually a dynamic equilibrium is established with the metal attaining a negative potential due to the excess of electrons. Different metals establish different negative potentials and the greater the negative potential, the greater the tendency to dissolve. The potential developed is referred to as the electrode potential. The electrode potentials of all metals are normally listed in order of magnitude and the list is referred to as the electro-chemical series. Useful facts of this series are that it gives an indication of the relative corrodability of metals and explains why two dissimilar metals in electrical contact and immersed in an electrolyte will generate an electric current; in general, the metal with the higher negative potential will undergo dissolution.

For dissimilar metal corrosion to occur we require:

(a) One metal (anode) to dissolve and produce a continuous supply of electrons.
(b) The other metal (cathode) to provide a site for continuous electron removal.
(c) A reservoir to receive the ions produced by dissolution.
(d) An external electrical contact between the two metals.

The anode reaction has been given above. The cathode reaction will depend on the nature of the electrolyte. In neutral or alkaline solutions, the reaction to remove electrons depends on the amount of oxygen available. If the oxygen supply is plentiful, then the following occurs:

$$O_2 + 4H_2O + 4e \rightarrow 4OH^-$$

If the supply is limited, the reaction is:

$$O_2 + 2H_2O \rightarrow H_2 + 2OH^-$$

It is not necessary to have two different metals to produce an electrochemical action; anodes and cathodes may be produced on a single metal surface if the latter is non-homogeneous. Non-homogeneity may be produced by variations in grain size, residual strain, composition differences, etc.

A complicating factor in predicting which metal corrodes and the intensity of attack, is the presence or creation of chemical films on the metal surface. Such films isolate the metal from the electrolyte and slow down or stop metal ion loss. The effect is known as passivation and often the protective film is deliberately created on the metal by an electrochemical process prior to use. Whether or not passivation occurs will depend on the electrode potential and the solubilities of the films produced. This in turn depends on the pH of the electrolyte and any externally imposed potential. It is usual to plot such information on a special diagram called a Pousbaix diagram. Such a diagram will indicate those combinations of pH and potential which provide protection or promote dissolution. The diagrams are useful but give no indication of solution rates or the effect of the presence of additional ions in the electrolyte, e.g. chloride ions are known to promote breakdown of passive films. Extra information on the mechanical strength of films and their ability to repair damaged areas is also needed.

The fact that corrosion between unlike metals is electrochemical can provide means of protection. The second metal can be used to create and maintain a passive film on the major structural element — anodic protection.

Alternatively, the second metal may be chosen to dissolve preferentially and supply electrons to the main structural metal, thus rendering the normal corrosion mechanism impossible — cathodic protection. A problem with this technique is that to provide continuous protection requires continuous solution of the anode and the resulting products may be deleterious. For both anodic and cathodic forms of protection the relative surface areas are important. The most favourable combination being large anode/small cathode. This ensures uniform corrosion.

The passive film that certain metals develop and maintain allows them to be used in combination; alloys based on titanium mobium and tantalum possess this feature. This property is useful in that it enables designs that demand differing properties in different positions in the same artefact, to use different materials.

Additional corrosion mechanisms

In addition to the above there are several special types of corrosion which can occur. These are crevice corrosion, stress corrosion and corrosion fatigue.

Crevice corrosion

The importance of oxygen as an 'electron remover' has already been mentioned. It is also important in a form of corrosion called crevice corrosion. This arises when scratches are produced on metal surfaces or when artificial crevices are produced between metal joints. Oxygen supply to the electrolyte at the root of a crevice is limited by diffusion but that at the outer surface is good. Differences in oxygen concentration result in the area which receives more oxygen becoming cathodic to metal 'hidden' at the root of the crevice. The latter undergoes dissolution and the electrons produced are rapidly oxidized at the cathode. Deep penetration of the metal is possible and rapid strength reduction can occur.

Stress corrosion

The combination of a tensile stress plus corrosion is a particularly severe form of attack. Corrosion produces pits which act as stress concentrations. The presence of a tensile stress develops these pits into cracks which then suffer further attack by crevice corrosion. It may be avoided by proper alloy formulation.

Corrosion fatigue

The combination of cyclic loading plus corrosion leads to a situation where no fatigue limit exists. The action is similar to the above in that corrosion develops pits to act as stress concentrations and the tensile part of the load cycle serves to develop the pits into cracks.

Non-metallic corrosion

Information on the behaviour of non-metallics is less comprehensive than for metals. Characterization problems arise because of variations in polymerization and the presence of additives such as plasticizers, pigments, fillers, etc. Additives may initiate more reaction than in the pure polymer.

As yet no satisfactory accelerated corrosion tests exist and there is lack of information on rates of dissolution. Furthermore, no accepted mechanisms exist to describe effects of stress and chemical attack in combination or wear and corrosion.

Desirable properties in implant materials

The previous sections have described how an assessment of the differing properties of a material are made. The more difficult task is to establish which particular features are desirable in a particular application. In general the attributes required comprise a number of properties, the sum of which is difficult to define with any precision.

Tensile strength by itself has little significance. For example, aluminium alloy, nylon, mild steel, have comparable strengths but differ greatly in all other respects. Tensile strength of brittle materials is controlled by the number, size and location of cracks so that a particular value is of significance only if the scatter is known. Obviously sufficient strength must be available but it is surprising how low a value can be tolerated if other properties are satisfactory. Similar comments apply to stiffness and yield strength.

Toughness is probably the most important attribute of any structural material. However, brittle materials can be successfully employed under slow or static loadings and if used in compression. Ductility is related to toughness and is a desirable property if an implant has to be altered in shape, i.e. bent, at the time of implantation. Most implants are, however, used without alteration of shape and ductility is only an asset in its original manufacture. Care should be taken in selecting the amount of ductility for use with long-term implantation, it may lead to deformation. If the implant has to be removed, the deformation can inhibit removal.

Fatigue failure has become more frequent in implants with the increase in total joint replacement. It has been estimated that up to three million load cycles per year of hip or spine can occur and at this level fatigue is certainly possible. Probably implant geometry has greater influence than material properties for such applications.

Fatigue failure is often associated with poor design, workmanship or handling. Elimination of stress concentrations such as sharp changes of cross-section would increase fatigue life. However, surface damage during insertion can become the site of fatigue cracks. The behaviour of an implant will depend a great deal on the attention given to the positioning of fractured parts of the bone during fixation.

This has been demonstrated in bone plates, where inaccurate reconstruction of the adjacent bone (to enable it to carry some of the load) had led to premature failure.

For a large number of implants, the vexed question of what stiffness to employ remains a matter of controversy. For some applications, e.g. bone plates for the hand, the choice has to be a rigid material. However, for most bone-plate applications, the implant must not be so stiff as to limit the healing rate of the fracture nor must it be of a stiffness which will not give adequate support. One solution is to use the latter and limit the loads applied.

MATERIALS RANGE

There is now a vast range of materials available to an engineer. These range from soft ductile metals to hard brittle ceramics, plastics lying between the two. The range of moduli extends from 10^{-3} to 10^3 GN m^{-2}. Ceramics and hardened metals are at the top of the range. Polymers which are far more compliant are several orders of magnitude less stiff and lie at the bottom end. Similar comments apply to yield strength where the range is from about 0.1 MN m^{-2} to around 5×10^4 MN m^{-2} and tensile strength where the range is from 0.2 to around 5×10^4 MN m^{-2}. Sometimes weight of a component is an important factor and it is then useful to normalize properties to provide a realistic comparison. Normalization is achieved by dividing the property in question by the density to give what are termed specific properties.

While there exists a remarkable range of available materials it should be appreciated that only a few of these warrant serious consideration. The body is a highly corrosive environment and is often unable to tolerate the presence of minute concentrations of material that may be dissolved from an implant. Among the metallic materials those which merit consideration are materials based on iron, cobalt, nickel, titanium, tantalum, zirconium, silver, gold and platinum. Tantalum and noble metals do not have suitable mechanical properties for most orthopaedic applications and zirconium is too expensive. Among the non-metallic materials are the glasses, crystalline ceramics and carbon and the plastics materials (including composites). Glasses and ceramics suffer from brittleness, plastics have lower strengths, good ductility but the presence of additives must be considered. Composites are materials which try to imitate nature by the incorporation of strong fibres in the softer plastic matrix.

Metals for implantation

All the metals are used in alloy form; the alloy addition has a profound effect on structure and hence properties. The addition may completely dissolve or produce intermetallic compounds.

Steels

Iron forms the basis of a wide range of alloys and to understand what occurs on alloying we should first examine the properties of iron and the effect of the major alloy addition, carbon. Iron exhibits allotropy. Below 908°C it exists as a body-centred cubic structure, called ferrite. Above 908°C it changes its atomic pattern to the face-centred cubic structure, austenite, and at still higher temperatures it transforms to yet another allotrope. The addition of carbon to iron alters the allotropic transformation temperatures. The solubility of carbon in ferrite is less than 0.02% at ambient temperature but the solubility in austenite is approximately 2%. This means that for alloys with a %C greater than 0.02% the conversion of austenite to ferrite results in excess carbon being precipitated as a compound. The precipitation can be prevented by rapid cooling and this creates a metastable structure called martensite. This phase is much harder than either ferrite or austenite and is brittle. It is usually used to impart wear resistance and indentation resistance.

Stainless steels

The only ferrous alloys of practical importance in orthopaedic application are the stainless steels which are produced by alloying principally with chromium, nickel and carbon.

The principal effect of carbon is to increase strength and hardness but there is a consequent reduction in ductility. Strength properties can be increased further by heat treatment. When chromium is present it forms hard carbides which, because they deplete the iron matrix of chromium, will reduce corrosion resistance.

Chromium has a great resistance to corrosion which is attributed to formation of a dense resistant film of chromium oxide. It dissolves readily in iron and restricts the range within which austenite forms. Above 13% ferrite is the stable phase at all temperatures.

Nickel is always added to steels in conjunction with chromium, never alone. Nickel additives counter the grain coarsening effects of chromium. More importantly, it expands the range of austenite stability and hence permits the addition of larger amounts of chromium and also molybdenum. Both of these increase the strength and corrosion resistance. For surgical implants the only recommended alloys are the molybdenum-bearing austenite steels with 18–20% chromium and 10–14% nickel. Recommended alloys are included in Table 1.1. Currently nickel-based alloys are not used in orthopaedic

Table 1.1 — Typical properties of implant alloys

Alloy type	Mechanical properties				
	Yield strength (MN/m^2)	Tensile strength (MN/m^2)	Percentage elongation at fracture	Young's modulus (GN/m^2)	Hardness (Vickers)
316 Stainless steel in annealed condition	280	650	45	210	190
316 Stainless steel in cold-worked condition	750	1000	10	230	320
^{a}Cobalt chrome in cast condition	400	690	8	240	300
^{a}Cobalt chrome in cold-worked condition	400	1540	8	240	300
Pure titanium	470	710	30	120	310
Titanium 6% aluminium 4% vanadium as cast	970	1000	12	120	320

^{a}Trade names: Vitallium, Zimalloy, Protasul 2.

work but the inconels and nimonic range do have high corrosion and wear resistance and are potential materials.

Cobalt-based alloys

The principal alloying elements are chromium, carbon, molybdenum and tungsten. The main alloys used are Stellite 21 and 25. The former has a high work-hardening rate and is therefore difficult to machine and must be cast to shape: it needs extensive testing for presence of casting defects in every component. The latter is machinable and has the better mechanical properties but is less resistant to crevice corrosion. Both alloys are comparable in cost to stainless steels. A new alloy, Protasul 10, has higher strength toughness and corrosion resistance, is capable of being mechanically worked, but is much more expensive than stainless steels.

Titanium-based alloys
The principal implant alloy is titanium 6% aluminium 4% vanadium alloy. This may be easily welded and machined. Corrosion resistance is good but they have poor resistance to erosion. The latter makes them unsuitable for the bearing surfaces in total joint replacement.

Glasses
Glasses have not been used for orthopaedic surgery but are subject to considerable research because of their similarity with ceramics. Main interest lies in the biodegradable forms.

Ceramics
Essentially these are compounds of metals and non-metals which have high hardness and high temperature resistance. Principal drawback is brittleness and inability to cope with stress concentrations.

Plastics and composites
As with metals the vast majority of polymers are used in modified form. The combination of pure polymer plus additive is called a plastic. Typical additions are plasticizers to increase flexibility, ultraviolet light stabilizers, pigments, fillers and lubricants. For biomedical applications the additions are made to improve mechanical properties. Composites are plastics plus a reinforcing agent such as glass-fibre or Kevlar usually in fibre form. Modern synthetic composites imitate nature. The composites considerably increase strength without imparting too big a weight penalty and thus provide a high strength/weight ratio. The properties depend on the quantity of reinforcement added and it is possible to tailor these to the application. An attractive feature is the enhanced toughness of the composite.

HUMAN TISSUES AS MATERIALS

In any consideration of engineering in orthopaedic surgery, the structure and mechanical properties of the primary materials have to be examined. These primary materials are those which exist in the body itself. In the case of orthopaedics, these are bone and cartilage. A vast literature exists concerning the structure and properties of these two tissues and consequently only a comparatively limited synopsis of the salient features can be attempted here.

Cartilage

Cartilage is a phylogenetically ancient tissue. Its occurrence is widespread as both a temporary and permanent component of the skeleton and other body systems. In early life, a large proportion of the skeleton is composed of cartilage, much of which, in the course of time, is replace by bone. In the adult, cartilage persists in the walls of the thorax, trachea, larynx, ears, nose, bronchi and the articulating surfaces of the synovial joints. In the synovial joints, the articulating surface is modified to be smooth and wear resistant and is aided in this by the lubricating effect of the synovial fluid. In other areas of cartilage, the surface is invested with a fibrous perichondrium or abuts against bone.

In common with other connective tissues, cartilage consists of cells (chondrocytes) embedded in a matrix. The matrix, which is an amorphous ground substance, surrounds a meshwork of collagen or elastin fibres which vary in their density and deposition in different areas. The ground substance is a firm gel which stains positively with the periodic acid–Schiff reaction, metachromatically with toluidine blue and is basophilic in conventional histological preparations. It contains some lipid, a high proportion of mucoproteins and acid and neutral mucopolysaccharides. It is the molecular architecture of these mucopolysaccharides which has often been held to explain the compression-resisting capacity of cartilage, while its high tensile strength has been attributed to the properties of the contained collagen.

The cells of cartilage, the chondrocytes, reside in spaces termed lacunae which exist within the matrix. In the layers of cartilage immediately beneath the perichondrium or under the free surfaces of articular cartilage, the cells are flattened with their long axes lying parallel to the surface. Deeper in this tissue the cells are angular or rounded and tend to become more rounded with age. The chondrocytes tend to be clustered in groups, each group being the offspring of a single parent cell. These small clusters are known as isogenous cell groups or cell nests.

The nucleus of the chondrocyte is rounded or oval and may contain one to several nucleoli depending on species. There is a well developed Golgi apparatus, mitochondria, a variable amount of rough endoplasmic reticulum, lipid deposits and glycogen.

In young tissue the Golgi and endoplasmic reticulum are prominent, but become less so in mature, quiescent cartilage.

The nutrition of cartilage

Cartilage is often described as an avascular tissue, i.e. a tissue which is not infiltrated by blood vessels. While this is not strictly true, it has to be said that the majority of chondrocytes are remote in relation to blood vessels. Nutrients pass to and from the cells along with metabolites by diffusion along concentration gradients across the intercelluar matrix. In the case of articular cartilage, the vessels are those of the synovial membrane and marrow cavity. Many cartilages are also penetrated by small branching canals which contain small blood vessels. The canals show a pattern of distribution which is fairly constant for a particular mass of cartilage. The timing of their appearance and disappearance may be quite variable. In the nasal and laryngeal cartilages they form in the seventh month *in utero* and persist until old age. In temporary cartilage, the canals appear in about the third month *in utero* and grow towards the site of the subsequent ossification centres. It has been suggested that they are formed as a direct preliminary to ossification, but this is probably not the case as their appearance in non-ossifying cartilage is also noted. Their main function is undoubtedly to provide nutritive support for the deeply placed cells in large, expanding masses of cartilage.

Histogenesis of cartilage

Histogenesis of cartilage is achieved by the transformation of embryonic mesenchyme. The mesenchyme cells condense, lose their irregular surface projections and become rounded. These cells soon become surrounded by a fine meshwork of collagen fibrils and associated chondromucoproteins which have been secreted by the cells themselves. Continued secretion of matrix and fibrils causes the cells to be pushed further apart until the typical structure of cartilage becomes recognizable.

In some circumstances, the matrix becomes laden with collagen or elastin fibres depending on the type of cartilage being formed. Subsequently, growth of a mass of cartilage occurs. This growth is both interstitial and appositional.

Growth of cartilage

Interstitial growth occurs as a result of the frequent and continued mitotic division of the early chondroblasts throughout the thickness of the tissue mass. When a cell divides the resulting daughter cells both occupy the same lacuna but are soon separated by a wall of matrix deposited between them which is gradually thickened, resulting in the separation of the cells. Interstitial growth is prominent only in young cartilage where there is sufficient plasticity in the matrix to allow continued expansion from within.

Appositional growth occurs as a result of proliferation of cells of the inner chondrogenic layer of the perichondrium. Some of the resultant cells differentiate into chondroblasts which are deposited on the outer surface of the cartilage. These cells then secrete a layer of matrix and become embedded in their own lacuna. The process of adding new chondroblasts is repeated, while those more recently established within their own lacuna divide and add more cartilage by interstitial growth.

Cartilage is usually classified according to the fibres which are contained within the matrix. The classifications are hyaline cartilage (hyalos meaning glass), white fibrocartilage (containing much collagen) and yellow elastic fibrocartillage (containing a rich elastin network).

Hyaline cartilage

Hyhaline cartilage is a widespread tissue during embryonic life as it provides the basis for the ossification of the greater part of the skeleton. In the adult it persists in the larynx, trachea, bronchi, the costal cartilages and the articular cartilages. The interstitial matrix of hyaline cartilage contains an extremely fine meshwork of collagenous fibrils which are arranged in a characteristic pattern with reference to the isogenous cell groups and to the mechanical requirements of the tissue mass as a whole.

White fibro-cartilage

This type of cartilage consists usually of little more than dense white fibrous tissue with small scattered islands of cartilage cells. When present in bulk, as in the intervertebral discs, it provides a tissue of great tensile strength combined with an appreciable degree of elasticity. In areas where it is present in lesser quantities, such as the glenoidal and acetabula labra and the cartilaginous lining of the long grooves which accommodate tendons, it is a tissue of great toughness and sufficient elasticity to enable it to resist long-term pressure and friction. The articular surfaces of membrane bones such as the mandible and clavicle are also invested with white fibrocartilage.

Yellow elastic fibrocartilage

In elastic cartilage the matrix is permeated with a rich network of elastin fibres which provide the tissue with considerable resilience. This type of cartilage occurs in a few isolated regions in man; these include the external ear, the corniculate cartilages of the larynx, the epiglottis and the apices of the arytenoids. In contrast to hyaline cartilage it exhibits much less tendency to calcify with advancing age.

The mechanical properties of cartilage

The two mechanical functions of articular cartilage are to distribute weight and to provide a bearing surface. The directional nature of the structure of cartilage suggests that the mechanical properties will vary with direction, i.e. that the material is anisotropic and the presence of an hydrated gel and free water in the matrix suggests that the mechanical properties will be time dependent.

Bone

Bone, in common with other connective tissue, consists of cells, fibres and ground substance, but bone is unique in that its extracellular components are calcified making it a hard, stiff substance ideally suited for its supportive and protective function in the skeleton. Bone is a dynamic, living material, constantly being renewed and remodelled in response to external mechanical stimuli.

In addition to the mechanical functions, bone plays a vital metabolic role as a store of ions which can be drawn upon as needed in the homeostatic regulation of the concentration of calcium and phosphates in the blood and other body fluids.

The major constituents of bone

Collagen

Collagen is the primary organic component of bone. It occurs in most tissues and is probably the most commonly occurring protein in the body. The amino acid sequence is so characteristic that it is almost diagnostic of collagen. The structure which this sequence forms is a slow left-handed helix referred to as a tropocollagen molecule. In order to form a fibre, the collagen molecules have to form a continuous structure with many overlaps to allow stresses to be transferred from one molecule to the next. A number of different types of collagen have been identified from different sources, the type occurring in bone being type 1. If examined in the transmission electron microscope, collagen is observed to have a regular banding pattern. The periodicity of this pattern is found to be 67 nm depending on the source of the collagen in question. The individual tropocollagen molecules are 280 nm long and are packed together in a regular form, although the exact nature of this packing still remains uncertain.

Mineral

The inorganic component of bone has long been recognized as being closely related crystallographically to mineral apatites. It has been more specifically identified as an apatite of calcium and phosphate which gives an x-ray diffraction pattern similar to the mineral hydroxyapatite which has the chemical formula $3Ca_3(PO_4)_2CaOH_2$. There are, however, many anions and cations associated with the crystal lattice, and despite years of research and many hundreds of publications, the exact nature of its crystallographic structure remains uncertain.

The cells of bone

The osteocytes

These are the living cells in bone tissue, they vary in number, spatial arrangement and appearance. They are most numerous in young bone and they conform to the general shape of the lacunae in which they lie.

Their processes which pass through channels termed canaliculi may be of considerable length and may also branch. Although these cellular processes meet those of other cells they are not continuous and terminate in end-to-end or side-to-side juxtaposition without any special junctions. The cytoplasm of the cell processes contains no distinctive organelles but a few smooth-walled vesicles and electron-dense granules are present.

The cell bodies of mature, relatively quiescent osteocytes contain an oval nucleus surrounded by a fairly small volume of basophilic cytoplasm. There is a correspondingly small concentration of rough endoplasmic reticulum, some free ribosomes, centrioles and a small juxtanuclear Golgi apparatus.

Neither the cell bodies of the osteocytes nor their processes fully occupy the lacunae or canaliculi in which they reside; a space, presumably fluid filled, surrounds them. There is thus a continuous extracellular space from the Haversian canals via the canaliculi and the lacunae through which the osteocytes are nourished and ion transport may be achieved.

The osteoblasts

Osteoblasts are the cells associated with the formation of osseous tissue and are invariably found on the advancing surfaces of developing or growing bone. They are usually between 20 and 30 μm in diameter. During active deposition of new bone matrix, they form a layer of cells connected to one another by short slender processes.

The nucleus is often at the end of the cell furthest from the bone surface. The cells contain well developed Golgi apparatus, numerous elongated mitochondria and give a strong histochemical reaction for alkaline phosphatase. When active bone formation ceases, the osteoblasts revert to a spindle shape and the phosphate reaction of the cells rapidly declines. Many osteoblasts become entrapped in their own secretions and consequently become osteocytes.

The osteoclasts

Closely associated with areas of bone resorption are the osteoclasts. They are giant cells with a variable number of nuclei, often as many as 15 or 20. They are frequently found in concavities in the surface of bone termed Howship's lacunae. During the reformation of the trabeculae of spongy bone in rapid growth, they are commonly seen enveloping the tip of each spicule of bone undergoing resorption. The nuclei resemble those of osteoblasts and osteocytes. The cytoplasm is slightly basophilic and often appears vacuolated. On the side adjacent to the bone, the cytoplasm may have a faintly striated appearance and there appears to be an infolding of the cell membrane forming a large number of irregularly-shaped lobopodia separated by narrow extracellular clefts. Observations of osteoclasts in tissue culture have demonstrated that this is not a stable surface feature but is highly active and constantly changes its configuration.

The mechanical functions and properties of bone

The most obvious mechanical functions of bone are those of the protection of vital organs (e.g. the ribs and skull), to act as levers for locomotion and to provide attachments for ligaments and tendons via which the muscles may act. As the mechanical properties of materials are dependent on their structure, let us first consider the structure of bone.

The macrostructure of bone

If a limb bone such as the femur is sectioned horizontally at its midpoint, the shaft or diaphysis is seen to be a tubular structure with walls composed of dense compact bone (*substantia compacta*) surrounding a central cavity — the medullary or marrow cavity. In life the latter contains the bone marow. At the proximal and distal ends of the shaft are the epiphyses. These consist mainly of spongy bone (*substantia spongiosa*) covered by a thin peripheral cortex of compact bone. Spongy bone consists of a three-dimensional lattice of branching spicules or trabeculae forming a labyrinthine system of intercommunicating spaces. In the adult these intercommunicating spaces containing the marrow are directly continuous with the marrow cavity of the diaphysis. (See Fig. 1.10.)

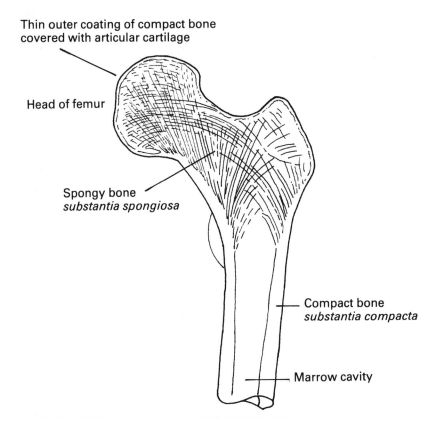

Thin outer coating of compact bone covered with articular cartilage

Head of femur

Spongy bone *substantia spongiosa*

Compact bone *substantia compacta*

Marrow cavity

Fig. 1.10 — Diagram of section through the head of the human femur and the distal portion of the diaphysis.

During growth and development, the epiphyses and diaphysis are separated by the cartilaginous epiphyseal plate, which is united with the diaphysis by columns of spongy bone in a transitional region called the metaphysis. The epiphyseal cartilage and the adjacent spongy bone of the metaphysis constitute a growth zone, in which increment in length occurs. On the articular surfaces of the epiphyses of long bones, the thin cortical layer of compact bone is invested with a covering of hyaline cartilage, the articular cartilage. The non-articular surfaces of bones are invested with a tough membrane, the periosteum, which has osteogenic capabilities.

The microstructure of bone

In the adult, compact bone consists mainly of a number of irregularly cylindrical units termed Haversian systems or secondary osteons, each consisting of a central Haversian canal which contains a neuro-vascular bundle and is surrounded by concentric lamellae of bony tissue. Within these lamellae are a number of lacunae which are connected with each other and with the Haversian canal by a number of fine radiating channels termed the canaliculi. The lacunae and canaliculi contain respectively the cell bodies and fine cytoplasmic extensions of the bone cells or osteocytes. The Haversian systems have a predominantly longitudinal orientation, with their long axes roughly parallel to the long axis of the bone; they do, however, frequently spiral, branch and intercommunicate. In transverse section they may appear round, oval or ellipsoidal and may vary considerably in diameter usually being between 50 to 200 μm across. The contained Haversian canals may also vary in diameter, with those closer to the marrow cavity being larger than average. Contained within each canal are one or two vascular capillaries and nerve fibres, the former transporting metabolites and waste products to and from the tissue via the blood.

The Haversian canals communicate with the free surface of the long bone, the central medullary cavity and each other via transverse channels known as Volkmann's canals. These differ from Haversian canals in that they are not surrounded by concentrically arranged lamellae but traverse the bone in a direction perpendicular or oblique to the long axis of the bone. The outer limits of each Haversian system is demarked by a cement or reversal line which indicates the limit of resorption which occurred prior to the formation of that Haversian system. The angular intervals between the Haversian systems are occupied by interstitial bone, which is made up of the remnants of woven bone, primary osteons, circumferential lamellae and older secondary osteons which have themselves been partly remodelled. The outer surface of long bones are encircled by other lamellae termed circumferential lamellae which are deposited under the periosteum during increase in girth of the bone.

The spatial arrangement of the collagen fibres
The nature of the lamellation observed in Haversian systems has long
been a topic of investigation. A number of hypotheses have been put
forward to explain the observed structure. It is not proposed to
examine these hypotheses in depth, but to give a brief outline of each
of the major options as follows:

(1) Fibre rich, mineral poor lamellae alternate with mineral rich,
    fibre poor lamellae.
(2) Each lamellae contains the fibres and mineral in the same
    proportions as its neighbours, the fibre direction, however,
    changes through approximately 90° from one lamella to the next.
(3) A combination of (1) and (2) above, where fibre rich, mineral
    poor lamellae alternate with mineral rich, fibre poor lamellae
    with the fibre orientation changing through 90° from one lamella
    to the next.
(4) Some Haversian systems have lamellae in which all the fibres in
    each lamella lie parallel to the long axis of the canal, while other
    Haversian systems contain lamellae in which the fibres are
    orientated circumferentially in each lamella. The direction of the
    fibre orientation being determined by the mechanical stresses to
    which the Haversian system in question is being subjected.

Options (2) and (4) above have been supported by a significant
body of research data. The picture, however, is by no means clear and
while the current research finding of one of the present authors would
favour option (2), it is acknowledged that this question is far from
resolved.

The ultrastructure of bone
Early investigations involving x-ray diffraction and transmission
electron microscopy of thinly sectioned bone suggested the presence
of a variety of needle- and plate-shaped hydroxyapatite crystallites
with dimensions varying between $\cong 2$ nm and $\cong 150$ nm. A number of
more recent investigations have suggested a model in which 'spheroidal'-shaped particles approximately 100 nm in diameter aggregate to
form a continuous mineral network which occupies the space
between the bundles of collagen fibres. This more recent view,
suggesting a continuous mineral phase which exists largely independent of the collagen, is more in keeping with the observed mechanical
properties of bone but as yet remains largely unaccepted.

The mechanical properties of bone

Over the last few decades, a large literature has built up on the mechanical properties of bone. Fortunately, there is a reasonable degree of agreement about most of these properties. The mechanical properties of interest in this case are elastic properties (Young's modulus) and strength (in tension, compression and shear).

Elastic properties

The elastic properties of bone may be measured in two ways:

(a) by applying a known load to a specimen, observing the resulting deformation and calculating the elastic properties, and
(b) by measuring the velocity of the propagation of sound in bone.

The velocity of propagation of sound in a medium is obtained from $V = \sqrt{(E/p)}$, where E is Young's modulus and p is the density of the medium. Measurements using the propagation of sound are much less straightforward than mechanical testing and consequently most of the published data are derived from direct loading experiments.

Strength of bone

The strength of a material is fairly easy to measure. The load at which the specimen breaks can be measured and the strength calculated directly. The figures for bone vary depending on the source of the sample tested but are of the order of 70–140 MN m^{-2} in tension and 140–210 MN m^{-2} in compression.

FURTHER READING

Crawford, R. C. *Plastics Engineering*, Pergamon Press, 1981.

Gordon, J. E. *Structures*, Pelican Books, 1978.

Kingery, W. D. *Introduction to Ceramics*, John Wiley, New York, 1960.

Landsdown, A. and Price, A. *Materials to Resist Wear*, Pergamon Press, 1975.

Materials Selector and Design Guide, Design Engineering, Morgan Grampian Publishing, London.

Scully, J. C. *The Fundamentals of Corrosion*, Pergamon Press, 1975.

Van Vlack, L. H. *Physical Ceramics for Engineers*, Addison-Wesley, Reading, MA, 1964.

2

Engineering theory

J. Richards

INTRODUCTION

This chapter explains, in simple terminology, basic engineering principles. This includes statics, stress, strain, bending and torsion.

Statics is the study of the external effects of forces and force systems on a body. Forces applied to an elastic medium results in a stress in the material. A function of stress is strain which is a measure of the change in geometry of a component. Bending moments produce changes in curvature while twisting deformation is described as torsion.

Each subject is explained with minimal mathematical theorem and abundant graphical representation.

STATICS AND DEFORMATION OF ELASTIC BODIES

Statics

This is the study of the external effects of forces and force systems on a body (component). These forces produce deformations in all materials (which are not 'rigid'). Force is a vector, having magnitude, direction and position (Fig. 2.1), and can be considered as the resultant of two or more components. Thus, AB is a force which is the resultant of two components AC and AD. The magnitude and direction of the force is determined from its components by the polygon (parallelogram) of forces; the components are derived from the resultant by the technique of resolution. The components AC and AD (Fig. 2.2) are inclined at 90° to each other, and AC is inclined at

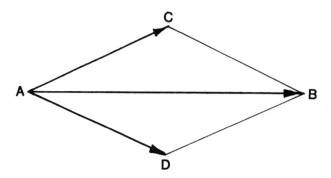

Fig. 2.1 — Simple vector diagram for two-force system.

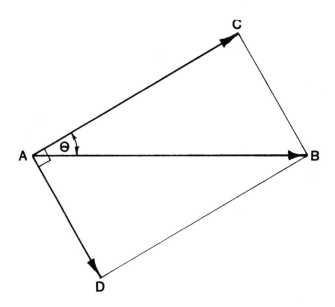

Fig. 2.2 — Resolution of a single force into two components.

an angle θ to the resultant AB. Then the components AC and AD are related to AB by simple trigonometry, and

$$AC = AB \cos \theta$$

$$AD = AB \sin \theta$$

A body in equilibrium has zero resultant force acting on it and the resolution of components in any direction is also zero. Consider the case of applied traction (Fig. 2.3), then the pulley A, connected to the limb will roll on the support wire until equal angles are subtended by *BA* and *CA* to the connecting link *AD*. This is necessitated since there will be equal tensions in the wire either side of the pulley A. The vector diagram (Fig. 2.4) shows the force system acting on the pulley A, which will be in equilibrium.

Equilibrium is also characterized by zero rotation, implying zero moment of forces. The moment of a force about a point is a measure of the rotational effect produced by the force, and is determined by the product of the force and the perpendicular distance measured from the point to the line of action of the force. The units for moment are those of force times distance, i.e. Nm, kNmm, etc. The moment required at the elbow, to support (not lift) a mass 5 kg in the hand, distance 250 mm from the elbow joint, will be $5 \times 9.81 \times 250$ Nmm (Fig. 2.5).

Forces arise from external agencies, body forces (gravity), friction and motion. It is not always necessary to analyse the entire system but only a portion of it — this is referred to as the free-body diagram — it is the basic tool in solving biomechanical problems. Consider the forces acting on the lower limb with a person standing on that leg only. The forces acting on that limb only represent the free-body diagram (Fig. 2.6). The relevant forces are: the mass of the limb, ω, the reaction on the foot by the ground surface, W, the reaction Q at the head of the femur (assumed to act through the centre of rotation) and the force P due to the abductor muscle. The forces P and Q are replaced by the components P_x and P_y, Q_x and Q_y respectively in directions parallel and perpendicular to ω and W (Fig. 2.7). Then resolving horizontally:

$$P_x = Q_x$$

and resolving vertically:

$$Q_y + \omega + W - P_y = 0$$

where

$$P_x = P \cos \alpha, \quad P_y = P \sin \alpha$$

$$Q_x = Q \cos \beta, \quad Q_y = Q \sin \beta$$

The behaviour of the femoral head during single stance phase of gait can be examined by considering the free-body diagram of that part of the body less the weight of the limb below the femoral head. The moment of the forces is considered about the centre of rotation (Fig. 2.8) whence for equilibrium:

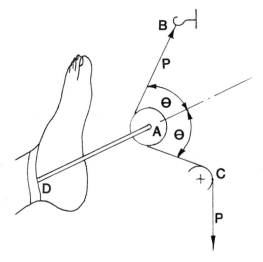

Fig. 2.3 — Application of vectors in traction.

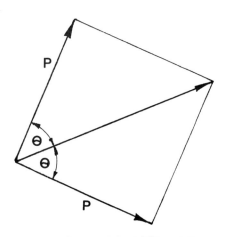

Fig. 2.4 — Vector diagram for combination of forces in Fig. 2.3.

$$P.C=W.b$$

b and c being estimated distances from the centre of mass of the part body weight and the abductor muscle to the centre of rotation, respectively. Essentially it is necessary to establish two independent equations to solve for the two unknowns, P and Q. The force Q is an

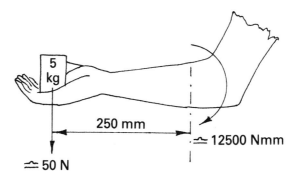

5
kg

250 mm

≃ 12500 Nmm

≃ 50 N

Fig. 2.5 — Representation of moments in equilibrium.

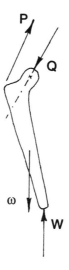

P

Q

ω

W

Fig. 2.6 — Free-body diagram (resultant forces) for the femur.

idealized force on the femoral head which is distributed in a non-uniform manner (Fig. 2.9), which is further modified during malfunction.

STRESS

Forces and force systems (couples) applied to an elastic medium result in a stress in the material. Stress is a measure of the resistance to deformation and is an internal condition within the material atomic

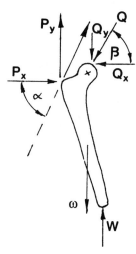

Fig. 2.7 — Component forces at the upper end of the femur.

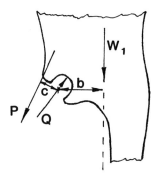

Fig. 2.8 — Single stance gait — resultant forces.

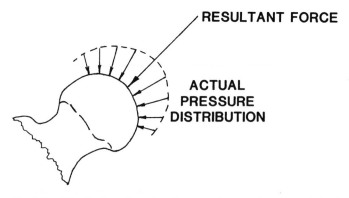

Fig. 2.9 — Distribution of pressure (compressive stress) on femoral head.

structure. It is an indication of the onset of elastic failure and ultimate collapse — it is measured by the resisting force per unit area (Nm^{-2}). Stress need not be, and is generally not, uniform; it may vary from point to point within a material so that we have the concept of stress at a point as the resistance in a prescribed direction or on a prescribed plane (surface) passing through the point. A stress $200\,Nmm^{-2}$ implies that on a surface of area $10^{-3}\,mm^2$ there is a resistance of $200\times10^{-3}\,N$, so that whereas the actual resisting force may change with the significant area, the stress is specific. Stress measured normal (perpendicular) to a surface or plane is described as tensile or compressive (symbol σ); stress parallel or tangential to a plane is shear (symbol τ) (Fig. 2.10). If either type of stress (normal or shear)

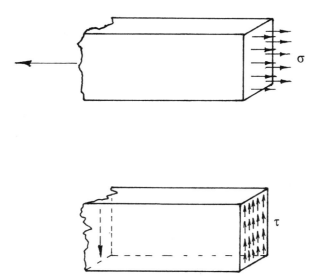

Fig. 2.10 — Representation of (a) tensile (normal) stress (b) shearing stress.

is present without the other then this is described as simple stress on that particular surface. The stress at a point can be defined in an infinite number of possibilities dependent upon the specified direction, thus in the case of a simple tensile force, the variation of stress (tensile and shear) at a point is shown in the polar plot (Fig. 2.11) from which it is seen that the maximum tensile stress is in the direction of the force and given by force divided by cross-sectioned area; there will be shearing stress reaching a maximum value at an

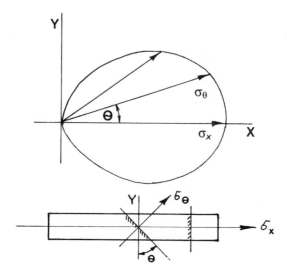

Fig. 2.11 — Polar representation of stress at a point.

angle 45° to the direction of the load. It is a condition of uniform stress that the external force producing the stress is applied through the centroid (centre of area) of the cross-section.

STRAIN

Since all materials are deformable, the measure of deformation, strain, is a function of stress. Strain is a measure of the change in geometry of a component (or element of a component if the strain is variable). Linear strain is associated with the change in length of the side of a component. This strain may be in the direction of stress or in a prescribed orientation relative to it. Angular deformation is described by the shearing stress (Fig. 2.12). Strain is a non-dimensional parameter and is related to displacements or movements which occur in the stressed material. Linear strain is represented by the fractional change in length of a prescribed 'gauge length'; shear strain is measured (radian) by the change in a right-angled corner of an element. Strains can be combined, when combined stresses are present (Fig. 2.13).

Engineering materials exhibit strains of the order 1% at the elastic limit; biological materials range from 2 to 100 per cent (soft tissue). Within the elastic limit, stress and strain are related to the proportionality law of elasticity (Hooke). The gradient of the stress/strain characteristic is a measure of the 'stiffness' of the material and is

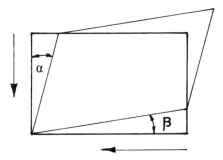

Shear Strain, $\phi = \alpha + \beta$ radian

Fig. 2.12 — Shear distortion — shear strain.

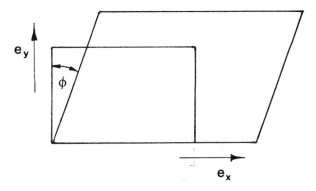

Fig. 2.13 — Composite strain — normal and shear strains.

called the modulus. Tensile and compressive effects are related by Young's modulus, E; shear stress and strain by the modulus of rigidity, G; the bulk (hydrostatic, fluid) stress and strain by the bulk modulus, K.

Stress is also associated with strain, or movement, or prevented movement. Thus a tensile force produces elongation in its own direction, while simultaneously in directions perpendicular to the direction of the force there will be a reduction in size (Fig. 2.14). Thus a strain can occur in a direction in which the stress is zero. The strain in a given direction will be the superposition of the components due to direct stress and the components due to lateral stresses. The axial

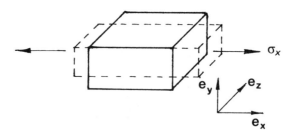

Fig. 2.14 — Direct stress introducing longitudinal and lateral strains.

(longitudinal) strain is related to the lateral strain (due to the same stress by a constant (for a given material). The ratio:

lateral strain/longitudinal strain = −Poisson's ratio (ν)

the negative sign implying an opposite type of displacement. Typical values for Poisson's ratio are 0.25–0.33. In a simple (uniaxial) system of tensile stress, σ_x, the axial or longitudinal strain is given by the elastic relationship $e_x = \sigma_x/E$, and the lateral strains $e_y = e_z = -\nu(\sigma_x/E)$, i.e. $e_y = e_z = -\nu e_x$ where x, y and z are considered mutually perpendicular directions. In a general, three-dimensional system, σ_x, σ_y, σ_z, the strain comprises the superposition of terms similar to those above with contributions from each of the stress components influencing the resultant strains:

$$e_x = \sigma_x/E - \nu\sigma_y/E - \nu\sigma_z/E$$
$$e_y = \sigma_y/E - \nu\sigma_z/E - \nu\sigma_x/E$$
$$e_z = \sigma_z/E - \nu\sigma_x/E - \nu\sigma_y/E$$

Any complex stress system can be resolved into a *principal* stress system, such as x, y, x, where there is no shearing stress on the x, y, z planes. There will be only three such planes in any system — they are unique and contain the maximum, minimum and intermediate value, in algebraic terms, e.g. $\sigma_1 > \sigma_2 > \sigma_3$, where $\sigma_1 = 250$ units, $\sigma_2 = 0$, $\sigma_3 = -50$ units. Generally, the stress at a point will have an infinite number of different values according to the orientation, and a specific value is identified according to the particular property being examined, i.e. tensile, compressive or shear. A typical distribution at a point due to a single tensile force is shown in Fig. 2.15, indicating the maximum tensile stress in the direction of the force ($\sigma = P/A$) and maximum *shearing* stress (although a *tensile* force is applied) in directions 45° to the direction of force. Conversely, if a shearing stress

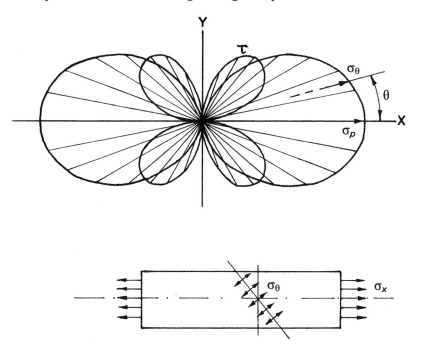

Fig. 2.15 — Stress components in various directions at a point.

is directly applied, it introduces tensile stresses at 45° to the direction of shear — explaining the tensile failure of some brittle materials when subjected to torsion (twisting, shear).

EXPERIMENTAL METHODS

It is difficult to measure stress since it represents interatomic bonding at crystal boundaries or transcrystalline strength. Strain measurement poses the problem of measuring small displacements or distortions — it is generally easier to measure linear strain and derive angular measure from it. The problem of small magnitude is overcome by using instruments or material having a high sensitivity and resolution. Methods in common use include electrical, acoustic, pneumatic and optical — size is often a critical factor.

Experimental methods measure the average strain over a prescribed gauge length, and the stresses are obtained from constitutive equations using the elastic constants of modulus and Poisson's ratio. In the study of biomechanics, *in vivo,* the major contribution has come from work using electrical resistance strain gauges, either directly bonded or through a transducer (Fig. 2.16). The change in

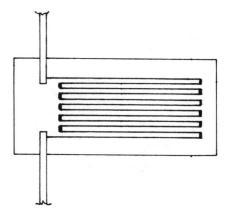

Fig. 2.16 — Typical wire grid electrical resistance strain gauge.

resistance is measured on a strain bridge, from which the stress is evaluated (Fig. 2.17). Since complex stresses often prevail, it is sometimes necessary to employ strain gauge rosettes and evaluate principal values (Fig. 2.18). The gauges in a rosette have a prescribed angular separation which is a parameter in the computational work. Strain gauge techniques require certain precautions to ensure sensible and accurate analysis. The features which require consideration include adequate temperature compensation, low loss connections to bridge, appropriate cement properties, identifications of stress gradients and concentrations. In cases where experimental methods are inadequate, it is necessary to resort to mathematical modelling and numerical methods which are outside the scope of this text.

STRAIN ENERGY

This describes the *state* of a stressed body (component). Energy is always a positive quantity and is independent of the type of stress (tensile, compressive, shear). In the case of uniform stress, the energy per unit volume (U) is given by:

$$U = \sigma^2/2E \text{ (tensile or compressive)} \quad \text{or} \quad \tau^2/2G \text{ (shear)}$$

It represents the external work done on the component to achieve this stressed state. If the work is gradually introduced then the stress is of the type $\sigma = P/A$, where P is the external force doing the work. In the case of impact, the energy (work done) is considerably greater and may often exceed the energy corresponding to the limit of

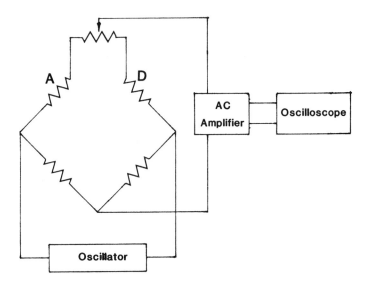

Fig. 2.17 — 4-Arm AC bridge circuit.

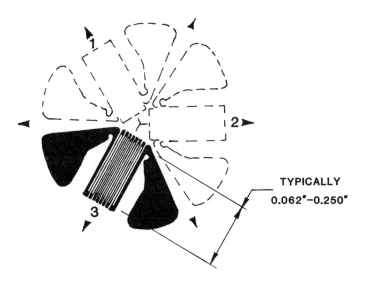

Fig. 2.18 — Equiangular foil-type strain gauge rosette.

elasticity — in which case the material fails. Thus a falling mass, weight W, is likely to cause failure, depending upon the height of fall, whereas the same mass applied gradually may impose a steady state stress within the elastic limit.

COMPOUND BARS (COUPLED SYSTEMS)

Where components are arranged symmetrically about the load axis (two-sided fixation) the assembly behaves as a compound bar which has stress in each element (fixator/bone) according to the simple analysis:

equilibrium $P_1 + P_2 = P$

(Fig. 2.19). Subscripts 1, 2, refer to the elements (bar/bone), and P

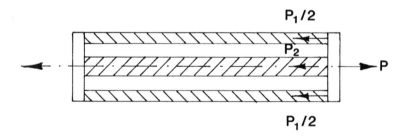

Fig. 2.19 — Simple compound bar with axial force.

would be the partial weight-bearing force.

Neglecting bending of the pins, the displacements/strains would be the same in the bone (callus) and fixator bars, thus:

$$e_1 = \frac{\sigma_1}{E_1}, \quad e_2 = \frac{\sigma_2}{E_2}; \quad e_1 = e_2$$

giving

$$\frac{\sigma_1}{\sigma_2} = \frac{E_1}{E_2}$$

and

$$\frac{P_1}{P_2} = \frac{\sigma_1 A_1}{\sigma_2 A_2} = \frac{E_1 A_1}{E_2 A_2}$$

describing the load sharing between callus and fixator. The analysis
can be developed in matrix form thus:

$$X_1 + X_2 = 0 \quad \text{(equilibrium, Fig. 2.20)}$$

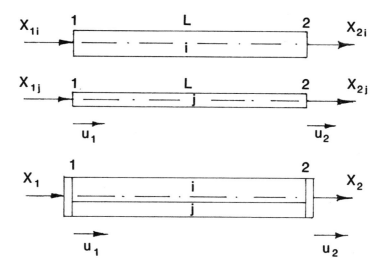

Fig. 2.20 — (a) Simple bar elements (2 nodes). (b) Coupled elements *i* and *j*
(compound bar).

where X_1 and X_2 are shown positive in the positive *x*-direction.
Displacements *u* occur at the *nodes* 1 and 2, then:

strain $= (u_1 - u_2)/L$

stress $= \text{strain} \times E = (E/L)(u_1 - u_2)$

axial force $= (AE/L)(u_1 - u_2)$

$$\left|\begin{matrix} X_1 \\ X_2 \end{matrix}\right|_i = \left(\frac{AE}{L}\right)_i \left|\begin{matrix} 1 & -1 \\ -1 & 1 \end{matrix}\right| \left|\begin{matrix} u_1 \\ u_2 \end{matrix}\right| \quad \begin{matrix} \text{(free-body diagram} \\ \text{— element } i) \end{matrix}$$

since

$$X_{1_i} = (AE/L)_i (u_1 - u_2)$$
$$\quad\quad\quad\quad\quad\quad\quad \text{(matrix multiplication)}$$
$$X_{2_j} = (AE/L)_i (u_1 - u_2)$$

and

$$X_{1_i} + X_{2_i} = 0$$

Combining elements i and j:

$$\begin{vmatrix} X_1 \\ X_2 \end{vmatrix} = \begin{vmatrix} X_{1_i} + X_{1_j} \\ X_{2_i} + X_{2_j} \end{vmatrix} = \begin{vmatrix} k_{11} & k_{12} \\ k_{21} & k_{22} \end{vmatrix} \begin{vmatrix} u_1 \\ u_2 \end{vmatrix}$$

where i can be the callus and j the fixator.

BENDING

Changes in curvature are produced by the effect known as the bending moment. Components are usually described as beams and the transverse loading of them produces bending. Associated with bending is a transverse shearing force. Stresses produced by bending moments are not uniform — the variation is due to two parameters, namely the magnitude of the bending moment and the position in the cross-section. The stress in a given cross-section varies from a maximum tensile, through zero to a maximum compressive (Fig. 2.21). The stress is zero at the neutral surface which coincides with

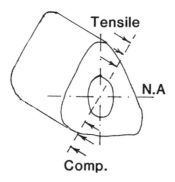

Fig. 2.21 — Distribution of simple bending stress in symmetrical bone section.

the centroidal axis in pure bending, i.e. no axial force. A beam will be held in a bent state under the action of bending moments (externally) and a moment of resistance (internally) which will be equal but of opposite signs for equilibrium. The beam section (Fig. 2.22) shows an

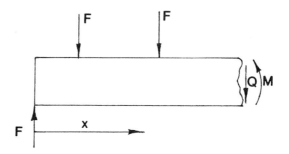

Fig. 2.22 — Presence of bending moments and shearing forces.

arrangement of forces (F) and the corresponding shearing resistance, Q, and moment of resistance, M, at a given cross-section. Equilibrium requires:

$$Q = \Sigma F$$

and

$$M = \Sigma Fx$$

The maximum stress occurs in a section where the bending moment is a maximum and the bending moment will be a function of loading and method of support. Examples of the distribution of moment due to a uniformly distributed load (UDL) are given in Fig. 2.23. The stress

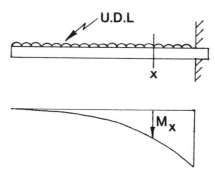

Fig. 2.23 — Bending of a cantilever with uniformly distributed load.

due to bending only is given in the form:

$$\sigma = My/I$$

where I is the second moment of area about the neutral axis and y the distance in the plane of the cross-section, measured from the neutral axis. Typical values of second moment of area (I) are given in Fig. 2.24 and a given section has two principal values (I), one being a

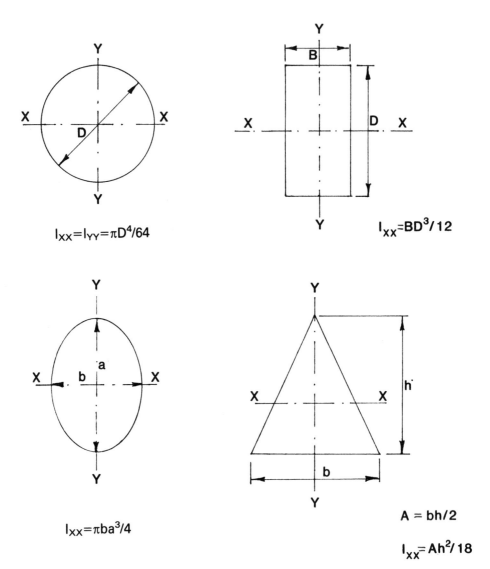

$$I_{XX} = I_{YY} = \pi D^4/64$$

$$I_{XX} = BD^3/12$$

$$I_{XX} = \pi ba^3/4$$

$$A = bh/2$$

$$I_{XX} = Ah^2/18$$

Fig. 2.24 — Geometrical properties of sections.

maximum and the other a minimum — (for a circle the principal values are equal). Where a section does not have an axis of symmetry, the principal axes have to be identified and the bending moment

·resolved in these directions. The tibia has principal axes approximately perpendicular to and parallel to a fixation plate. The behaviour of the tibia/plate combination will depend upon the sense of bending in relation to the principal axes, which are fixed. The product EI is called the flexural rigidity and, in the combination described, this factor will vary with the sense of bending, i.e. tending to open or close the fracture site; the range may be of the order of a factor 20.

Generally, the elements of the skeleton are rarely subjected to pure bending and the stresses are further complicated due to the non-uniform cross-section. Bending in the femur, for example, is due to a compressive load, applied eccentrically relative to the femur axis: Fig. 2.25. Stresses will be combinations of bending and direct loading, i.e. the superposition of M_0y/I and P/A, where M_0 is the product of eccentric force (P) and eccentricity (h) to femur axis.

TORSION

The twisting deformation is described as torsion and is the result of an applied turning moment about a longitudinal axis of a component — the twisting moment is called the torque. In the theory for circular solid or hollow cross-sections, a radial line in the section rotates to a new position due to torque and transverse sections remain plane after twisting, i.e. there is no warping of the section. The stresses due to torsion are shearing stresses, which are non-uniform in the cross-section. Torsional shearing stresses vary linearly across the section and are a maximum at the outside edge. The stress and the angle of twist are proportional to the applied torque and the simple stress relationship is $T/J = \tau/r = G\theta/L$ (Fig. 2.26). J is the second moment of area of the cross-section about the polar axis (axis of bar or tube), i.e. the axis about which rotation or twist occurs. The stress for a given torque is proportional to the factor r/J, and since J depends upon the fourth power of the diameter, significant increase in J can be introduced by small increases in outside diameter while material is removed at the smaller radius. Lightness and economic use of material is effected by the use of hollow sections, having strengths equivalent to that of a solid section with only small differences in external dimensions. Compound tubes can be analysed in a similar manner to compound bars, with shearing of torque according to geometry and elastic constant G.

The torsion of non-circular thin tubes is complex, but the concept of shear flow in the annulus is useful in understanding the behaviour (Fig. 2.27). In the case of thin tubes the flow will be parallel to the section boundary and the relationship can be written as $T = G\theta J^1/L$,

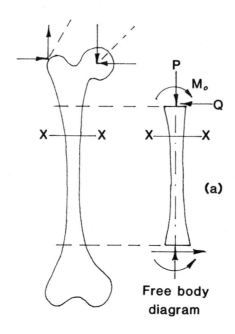

(a)

Free body
diagram

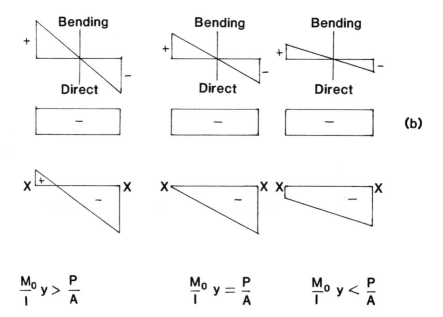

(b)

$$\frac{M_0}{I} y > \frac{P}{A} \qquad\qquad \frac{M_0}{I} y = \frac{P}{A} \qquad\qquad \frac{M_0}{I} y < \frac{P}{A}$$

Fig. 2.25 — Combined bending and direct stresses in a femur. (a) free body diagram,
(b) stress distribution.

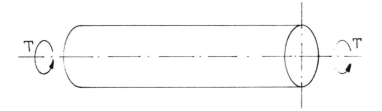

Fig. 2.26 — Twisting (torsion) in a bar of circular section.

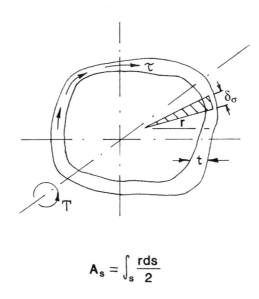

$$A_s = \int_s \frac{rds}{2}$$

Fig. 2.27 — Torsion in non-circular thin-walled sections.

where J^1 is the 'equivalent' second moment of area of the section about the axis of twist and is called the torsional constant.

The torsional stiffness of thin-walled open sections is considerably less than that for the closed tube, since the 'open' edge has no capacity to support a shearing stress (complementary) along the axis of the component. The continuity of the shear flow is interrupted, since the stress is zero at the free edge. Torsion of non-circular solid sections (square, triangular) is accompanied by warping of the section, i.e. non-planar behaviour. In the case of square or rectangular sections, the maximum shearing stress occurs at the mid-point of the side of the section — for the rectangle, the mid-point of the longer side, i.e. the point *nearest* the centre of twist.

STRUTS

Slender struts (length to diameter ratio greater than 30) are compression members which fail (elastically) due to a phenomenon or mode called 'buckling'. The maximum axial load which can be supported before the onset of instability is the buckling load. The diagrammatic representation of this critical stage is shown in Fig. 2.28, where the

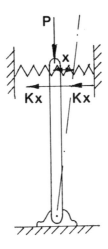

Fig. 2.28 — Critical condition with long member in compression.

elasticity of the compression member in the deflected state is shown as elastic springs, stiffness K. In the critical state:

$$Px=2KxL$$

The buckling load P is a function of K and L, where K includes geometry and modulus of material. The validity limit is often described in terms of a slenderness ratio parameter. The phenomenon is related to bending and again I, the second moment of area, is involved. If $I=A\times k^2$ where A is the cross-sectional area, then the slenderness ratio is L/k (hence the rough guide $L>30d$). The method of supporting the ends of the strut will modify the estimated buckling load and the behaviour of the strut subject to different end constraints is shown in Fig. 2.29.

Buckling is not usually a consideration when $L<30d$ and the struts are described as short and stocky. In these cases the end compressive load at the elastic limit is the simple product of stress and cross-sectional area. In the simple theory of buckling, it is assumed that the material is homogeneous, isotropic, the load is purely axial and applied through the centroid of the section, and that the strut is perfectly straight — these are ideal conditions which do not obtain in practice in the human skeleton.

BEARING LOADS

The treatment of contact between curved elastic bodies, such as joints and bearings, is associated with Hertz and often referred to as Hertzian stresses. In the case of a spherical ball and seating the contact surface is circular where the radius of the contact area depends upon the geometry of the bodies in contact and the elastic moduli of the bodies. The distribution of pressure is hemispherical (three-dimensional) and the maximum pressure is 1.5 times the mean — this assumes perfectly spheroidal surfaces; any deviation will considerably increase the stress levels.

STRESS CONCENTRATIONS

Stress analysis is often based on the assumptions of ideal conditions of geometry and loading, producing either uniform stress or gradual variation over a prescribed distance. However, in the vicinity of load or couple application or changes in component geometry, the maximum stress level will be higher than the mean by a stress concentration factor — this factor is often difficult to estimate. Typical geometrical conditions which give rise to stress concentration factors are notches, holes and screw threads. Small inclusions and imperfections in the structure of the material will have the same effect on the actual stress field.

Circular hole

For a small hole in a plate in tension or tube in torsion, the stress concentration factor $K_t=3.0$, the factor decreasing with increase in diameter of hole to width-of-plate ratio. In cases where the hole is in a component subjected to combined bending, torsion and direct load, the stresses are complex and the main observations are from experimental work.

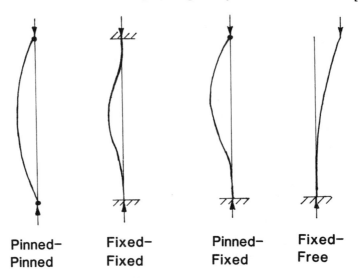

Pinned–
Pinned

Fixed–
Fixed

Pinned–
Fixed

Fixed–
Free

Fig. 2.29 — Types of end fixing in compression members.

Threads

Stress concentrations are significant where cyclic stresses are involved, causing premature failure due to fatigue. It is possible for the factor to reach levels of 10–12 at a distant one-third pitch from the bearing face of the screw — this can be reduced to 8–9 by careful design.

3

Surgical practice

I. G. Mackie, W. J. Mintowt-Czyz and L. D. M. Nokes

INTRODUCTION

This chapter presents the applications explained in Chapters 1 and 2 to orthopaedic situations. The mechanics of various bone fractures are analysed using engineering theorems which include stress and strain analysis. The process of fracture healing is briefly presented with its possible complications.

The latter half of the chapter includes orthotics which is the science of replacing missing parts of the human skeletal system. Methods of bone fracture management and the relevant engineering principles are explained which include internal and external bone fixation. Finally, a brief overview of hip and knee replacement is given.

FRACTURES

Bone fractures occur due to the application of a load. The type of fracture depends on the magnitude of the applied load, its direction and the bone itself. If the bone is weak due to some pathological condition, then the force required to fracture would be relatively smaller. To highlight the above principles, let us consider various parts of the skeletal system and how fractures may commonly occur.

Cervical spine

The cervical spine consists of seven vertebrae. The first two, C1 and C2, are specifically designed for flexion, extension and rotary motion. The C1 vertebra (Fig. 3.1) has large lateral masses that provide the only two weight-bearing articulations between the skull and vertebral

POSTERIOR

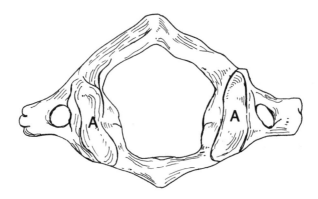

ANTERIOR

Fig. 3.1 — Superior view of the first cervical vertebra.

column. The second cervical vertebra (Fig. 3.2) provides rotation at its superior articulation with C1 and limited flexion, tilt and rotation at its inferior articulation with C3.

C3 to C7 vertebrae (Fig. 3.3) all have a similar appearance. They are structured to provide limited flexion, extension, tilt and rotation as well as stability to support the head. The bodies of the vertebrae articulate by intervertebral discs which are contained by the annulus fibrosis and the anterior and posterior longitudinal ligaments. The dense annulus fibrosis allows minimal movement between cervical spines.

In the cervical area, the spinal cord and its dural contents occupy approximately 50% of the spinal canal. At each intervertebral disc space, the ventral and dorsal rootlets join to form a nerve root which exits the spinal canal through the neural foramen.

Mechanisms of injury to the cervical spine
Excessive forces applied to the head in any direction may damage the bony and ligamentous complex of the cervical spine causing fractures, dislocations or both.

Forward flexion forces without axial load or rotation
Flexion at the facet joints and the discs is limited by the posterior ligamentous complex and the anterior and posterior longitudinal ligaments. Pure flexion generally results in no tearing of the ligamentous complex posteriority and no dislocation of the joints.

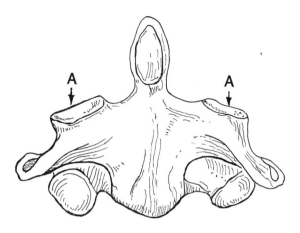

Fig. 3.2 — The second cervical vertebra.

Flexion-rotation forces

Rotation with flexion places unequal stresses on the posterior inter-spinous ligaments and facet joint capsules causing a unilateral facet dislocation. If the rotation-flexion forces are carried further, the opposite facet joint capsule tears resulting in a bilateral facet disloca-tion. This causes anterior subluxation of the intervertebral disc joint. Dislocations of the facets may be accompanied by fracture of the facet, lamina or vertebral body. The anterior longitudinal ligament is usually the only ligamentous structure that remains intact.

Axial load compression

Axial loads similar to those experienced when the head strikes an object in a diving position exert compressive forces on the midcervi-cal spine regardless of whether the head is flexed or extended. The force can result in comminuted fracture of the vertebral body, usually C5, being caught between C4 and C6. The posterior inferior margin of C5 vertebral body is frequently pushed into the spinal canal. The inferior disc between C5 and C6 is also frequently pushed posteriorly into the spinal canal. Severe neurological loss may result with quadriplegia.

Extension forces

The dorsal components of the cervical spine are well designed to limit hyperextension motion. The tough anterior and posterior longitudi-nal ligaments prevent distraction of the vertebral bodies anteriorly. Forces exceeding the normal extension range of the facet joint cause

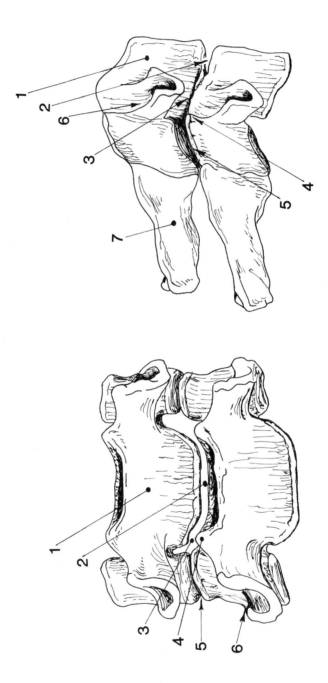

Fig. 3.3 — 1 Vertebral body, 2 disc, 3 uncovertebral joint, 4 uncinate process, 5 facet joint, 6 nerve root canal, 7 spinous processes.

the joints to lock in extension, and as the laminae and spinous processes touch, the force results in either fracture of the dorsal element by compression or in avulsion of the superior margin of the vertebral body by the anterior longitudinal ligament and annulus fibrosis. The spinal cord may be caught between the lamina and ligamentum flavum posteriorly and the bulge of the disc anteriorly resulting in severe neurological damage.

Lateral flexion

Lateral forces can cause compression on the lateral mass of the pedicles causing fracture of the masses. These rarely cause injury to the spinal cord.

Cervical injuries due to low or high velocity objects

Objects that strike the mid-cervical region at high velocity (3000 ft/s muzzle velocity) such as bullets usually cause complete spinal cord injuries. The injury usually involves gross instability due to the destruction of vertebral elements. Low-velocity (1000 or less ft/s muzzle velocity) objects cause less injury resulting in incomplete spinal cord damage.

Thoracolumbar spine

The thoracolumbar junction marks an abrupt transition between stiff and mobile segments. The lumbar spine is the second most mobile region. It is this mobility that makes the lumbar region more susceptible to fracture and dislocation if a force is applied that is sufficient to produce motion beyond the physiological range. The region from the twelfth thoracic vertebra to the second lumbar vertebra accounts for more than 50% of all vertebral body fractures. Motion in the thoracolumbar regions has six degrees of freedom (flexion, extension, right and left lateral bending, right and left torsion).

Typical thoracic and lumbar vertebrae are shown in Fig. 3.4. A lateral view of the spine is shown in Fig. 3.5. Each vertebra is attached to the adjacent vertebra by ligaments and is separated from each adjacent vertebra by intervertebral discs. The anterior longitudinal ligament is stronger than the narrow posterior longitudinal ligament. The anterior portion of the spine is well suited for bearing compressive forces and permits considerable motion around all degrees of freedom while also limiting translation. The intervertebral disc contains an avascular gelatinous nucleus bounded by the annulus fibrosis. Under compression the vertebral end-plates deform, forcing blood out of the cancellous bone through multiple vascular foramina

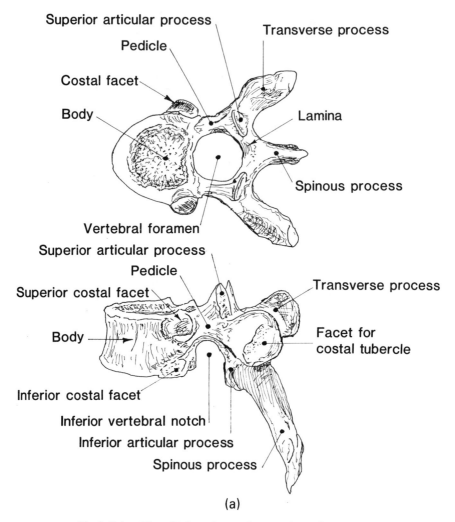

Fig. 3.4(a) — The mid-thoracic: vertebra superior and lateral view.

resulting in effective load damping. Also assisting damping is the intervertebral disc. Excessive compressive loading can result in fracture of the vertebral end-plates which allows the nucleus to invade the vertebral body. The vertebral end-plate always fails prior to annulus rupture in the normal spine (at a compressive load of approximately 230 kg).

The neural arch and vertebral body form a ring of bone that protects the dura and its contents. The neural arch with its associated processes, capsules and ligaments limits and controls the extent and direction of motion at each level. The neural arch is largely responsible for spinal stability.

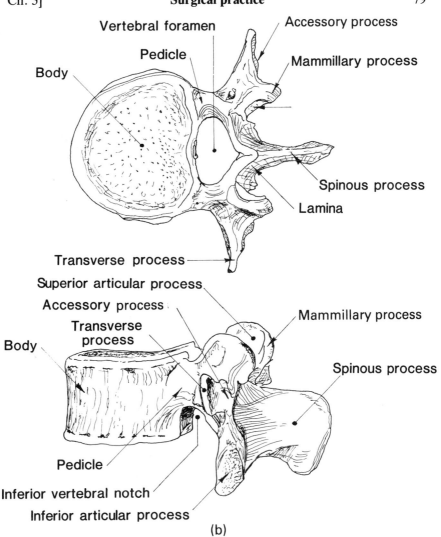

Fig. 3.4(b) — The mid-lumbar vertebra: superior and lateral view.

Pairs of ribs articulate with each thoracic vertebra at the level of the intervertebral disc. The thoracic cage permits ribs to function as stabilizers: restricting lateral bending, flexion and extension of the thoracic spine. The parallel arrangement of the ribs offers comparatively little restriction to torsion.

Mechanisms of injury to the thoracolumbar spine
Flexion (bending) fractures are the most common of all failure types, occurring most frequently at the thoracolumbar juntion. Flexion

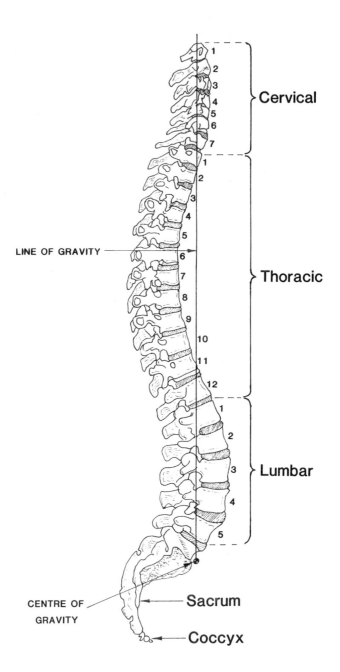

Fig. 3.5 — Lateral view of the vertebral column.

injuries are also seen at other areas of transition between stiff and mobile spinal areas such as the lumbosacral junction.

In the thoracic region, the distance between the flexion axis and the tip of the spinous process is three times greater than the distance between the axis and the anterior margin of the vertebral body. In the lumbar region, this ratio is 4:1. Therefore, when exposed to flexion loads, the anterior portion of the vertebral body experiences a compressive load that is three or four times greater than the tensile load experienced by the spinous process and supraspinous ligament. (Theory is discussed in Chapter 2.) For this reason hyperflexion produces a wedge-shaped fracture of the vertebral body.

Extension
In the thoracolumbar spine, extension fractures are quite rare. When they do occur, they are most often seen in the mid-lumbar region.

Lateral bending
Excessive lateral bending similar to hyperflexion produces a lateral wedge fracture due to asymmetrical loading on the vertebral body.

Rotation
A majority of rotational thoracolumbar fractures occur between T10 and L1. The lumbar spine has an inherently high torsional stiffness, due to the orientation of its facets. The region between T10 and L1 has relatively great rotational mobility. Therefore it is susceptible to those fractures in which torsion forces are important.

When the spine is exposed to combined rotation and flexion, the flexion component may produce a wedge fracture of the vertebral body. They may also yield a transverse translational displacement.

Shear
Transverse shear loads to the thoracolumbar spine produce translational unstable displacement of vertebra. There will be no evidence of rotational displacement or wedge-shaped fractures nor angular displacement.

Compression
Owing to its very high water content, an intact nucleus is not compressible under load. However, the adjacent cancellous bone is readily deformable and if loaded sufficiently it will fracture centrally producing an imprint of the adjacent non-compressible nucleus. Compressive fractures are the result of excessive vertical loading without flexion, rotation or lateral bending. They are most common in the mid-lumbar region. An effective crash restraint system, such as

a lap belt combined with shoulder harness, restricts angular displacement of the spine but favours the production of compression fractures.

Tension

When a wearer of a lap-type seat belt is subjected to sudden deceleration, his body is flexed over the restraining belt. All portions of the spinal column are posterior to the flexion axis; therefore the vertebral body is exposed to tensile stress. X-rays suggest that the vertebra are literally pulled apart, the most common site being between L1 and L4.

Spinal stability

Stability and instability are often applied to fractures and dislocations. A fracture or dislocation whose fragments are not likely to move during healing is generally considered to be stable.

A spinal fracture or dislocation is considered unstable if, during the healing phase, its fragments are capable of displacement that might produce neurological damage.

Pelvis

Fractures of the pelvis constitute 3% of all skeletal fractures. The pelvic girdle (Fig. 3.6) consists of two innominate bones which articulate anteriorly with each other at the pubis symphysis and posteriorly with the sacrum, which in turn articulates inferiorly·with the coccyx. Each innominate bone is made up of the ilium, ischium and pubis, all of which contribute to the formation of the acetabulum.

In the erect position, weight-bearing forces are transmitted from the upper femora to the acetabula and then through thick rings of the ilia called arcuate lines (Fig. 3.7). These lines meet the spinal column through the sacrum. This forms the femorosacral arch. This main arch is augmented by a subsidiary arch. The subsidiary arch is made up of the pubic bones and their horizontal rami.

In the sitting position, the weight-bearing forces are transmitted from the ischial tuberosities through the ilia and then into the sacroiliac joint (Fig. 3.8). This forms the ischiosacral arch. A subsidiary arch augments this main arch. The subsidiary arch is made up of the bodies of the pubic bones, the inferior pubic rami, and the ischial rami.

From a basic understanding of the force lines in the pelvis it is possible to speculate what type of fractures will occur under various stresses on the pelvis. Major fractures include those that involve the

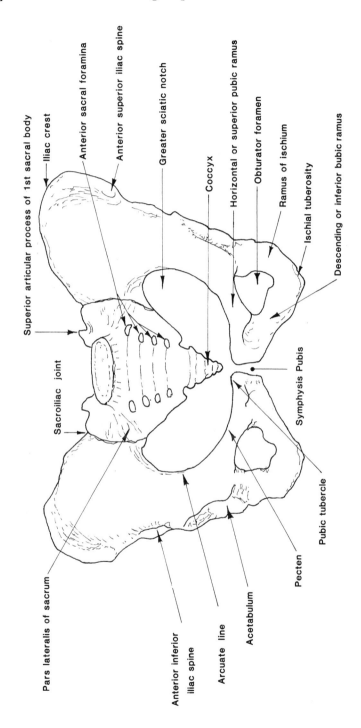

Fig. 3.6 — The pelvis.

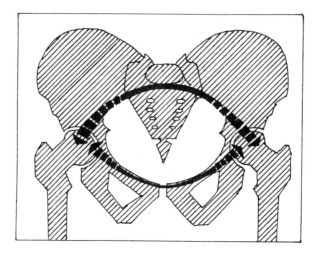

Fig. 3.7 — Diagram showing weight-bearing forces transmitted from the upper femora to the acetabular and then through the thick rings of the ilia (called the arcuate lines).

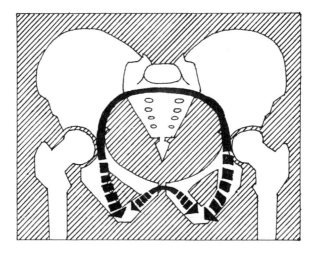

Fig. 3.8 — Showing the weight-bearing forces transmitted from the ischial tuberosities through ilia and then into the sacroiliac joints.

line of weight transmission from the spine to the acetabulum or, if they involve the rami, on both sides of the symphysis pubis. The remaining fractures of the pelvis are classified as minor.

Femur
Fractures of the femoral neck
The femoral head is not a perfect sphere. The joint between the pelvis and femoral head is only fully congruous in the weight-bearing position. The internal trabecular system of the femoral head is orientated along the lines of stress (Fig. 3.9) to which the bone is subjected.

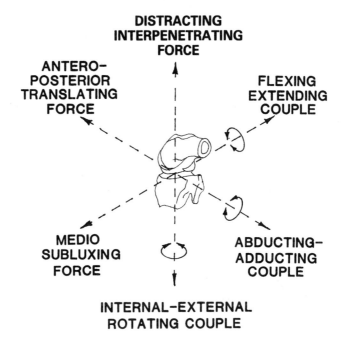

Fig. 3.9 — The force directions taken by the trabecular systems within the femoral head and neck.

Femoral neck fracture is rare in the young. Fractures may occur by direct forces or indirect forces such as levering the neck of the femur over the rim of the posterior acetabulum. Cyclical loading may produce micro and macro-torsional injury and falling may yield a complete femoral neck fracture. Muscles produce an axial load along the long axis of the femoral neck and coupled with external pressure, determine the fracture pattern.

Fractures of the shaft of the femur
The shaft of the femur is roughly tubular. Femoral shaft fractures usually result from major violence. In the young the wider metaphyseal areas frequently dissipate and transfer the stress force to other

areas of the femur. While the aged bone is somewhat more brittle and the resilience of the trabecular pattern is lost so that unacceptable stress forces more easily produce a fracture. Femoral shaft fractures are less common to persons in the older age groups, who usually suffer fractures of the metaphyseal ends of the long bone. The energy of impact may have been considerable resulting in multiple comminuted fractures.

Severe varus or valgus stress forces with axial loading and rotational forces produce the majority of the fractures in the distal femur. Most occur from high-velocity vehicle injury but falls from heights are also a frequent cause.

Tibia

Tibial shaft fractures are caused by direct violence to the tibia. High-energy injuries cause more open wounds, more loss of skin, more soft tissue damage and more bone displacement and comminution. Direct violence injuries are more likely to result in transverse or comminuted fracture lines, while oblique or spiral fractures are caused by indirect violence. Most indirect injuries result from recreational activities or falls. The foot may be anchored while the person falls, a torque is applied to the leg resulting in either a spiral or oblique fracture.

Other factors affecting fractures

A few examples have been given on how fractures may result. Any bone in the human body is capable of fracture if it receives sufficient stress. The point of fracture depends on the position, direction and magnitude of a force and also the strength of the bone at particular points. The cranial vault is likely to fracture along its suture lines on receiving a sufficiently high impact injury. The suture lines offer the least resistance to stress and hence act as propagating pathways for the lines of force.

Bone is a complex material which can orientate itself to carry maximum loading as highlighted in the trabecular pattern of the femoral neck. It is a living structure that can remodel itself to optimize changes in loading patterns. Pathological changes such as those associated with ageing will have profound effects on the mechanical properties of bone. The diseased bone will generally be relatively weak and more susceptible to stress fracture than its healthy counterpart.

Mechanical implants such as a hip prosthesis and internal fixation plates for fractures will also affect the properties of the bone. Although on the one hand strengthening the bone, it will cause changes in the dynamic modelling characteristics of the bone. The introduction of a screw thread into cortical bone can result in microfractures which, on application of a relatively small stress to the bone, yield a complete fracture. Implants can also weaken bone owing to the toxicity effects of either the implant material or the binding agent used to hold the prosthesis in place.

DEFORMITY

A deformity of any part of the body may be due either to abnormal bones, abnormal joints or a combination of the two. A deformity of a bone may be due to:

(1) Destruction or weakening of bones by disease.
(2) Injury to the bones.
(3) A disturbance of bone growth leading to an abnormal shape.

A deformity of a joint may be due to:

(1) Destruction or laxity of joint capsule.
(2) Scarring or fibrosis on one aspect of the joint capsule.
(3) Unequal muscle pull leading to contraction and possible dislocation.
(4) Displacement of the bone ends in relation to each other, e.g. as a consequence of misalignment of the articular surface, i.e. secondary to deformity of the bone.
(5) Traumatic displacement.

Deformity commonly involves both bone and joints.

Spinal deformities

An example of a combination of bone and joint deformities is often seen in spinal pathologies. The individual vertebrae are themselves distorted; the alignment of the articular surfaces is also distorted.

The mechanical or secondary deforming factors of the spine can be considered under the following headings:

(1) Gravity.
(2) The longitudinal fibres of the erector spinae muscle.
(3) The oblique (creep) fibres of the erector spinae muscle.

(4) The intercostal muscles.
(5) The abdominal muscles.
(6) The limb girdle (shoulder and hip) muscles.

Gravity

In the normally shaped spine in the upright position, the line of gravity runs from the external area downwards through the body of the fourth lumbar vertebra. The action of muscles, the shape of the vertebrae and the intervertebral discs and ligaments connecting the vertebrae resist collapse under the force of gravity. Once deformity has developed whether this be a lordosis, a kyphosis, a rotation or a lateral or rotation flexion, the force of gravity acts asymmetrically on the vertebrae and tends to increase whatever deformity is present.

Muscle action

The normal action of the longitudinal fibres of the erector spinae muscles is to extend the spine. Normally this extending action is balanced by gravity, length of the sternum and the action of the anterior abdominal muscles. If these factors are not operating, the forces exerted by the longitudinal fibres of the erector spinae muscle will be unopposed which would result in spinal deformity. The deep fibres of the erector spinae muscle run from one spinous process to the transverse processes of the vertebral bodies one, two or three segments below. If the lower vertebra is fixed then the action of, say, the right transverse spinal muscle, is to rotate the vertebrae above towards the opposite side (i.e. the left). If the left deep oblique fibres of the erector spinae muscle fibres are paralysed the tendency would be for the unparalysed right muscle to produce rotation of the vertebral bodies to the left. Once a rotation deformity has become established the muscles of the opposite side act at a mechanical advantage and this will tend to increase the deformity.

Intercostal muscles

Normally the heads of the ribs grip each thoracic vertebra as in a vice and their actions are equal. If the vertebral body is rotated the pressure of the heads of the ribs on the convex side is now posterior to the axis of rotation, but the pressure of the ribs on the concave side is anterior to the axis of rotation, i.e. the pressure of the heads of the ribs will act as a couple of forces and tend to increase the rotation. If deformity is established there will be a tendency to increase the rotation.

If a number of ribs are removed, the spine tends to deviate

towards the side from which the ribs have been removed. This shows that equal pressure of the ribs on the two sides of the spine is normally a factor in maintaining the spine in its straight position.

Abdominal muscles
The anterior or rectus abdominal muscles tend to increase kyphosis or diminish lumbar lordosis. If these muscles are paralysed a fixed lordatic deformity tends to occur. The lateral abdominal muscle and in particular the quadratus lumborum cause a convexity to the opposite side.

Limb girdle muscle
The psoas muscle tends to pull the vertebral bodies forwards on the same side. If a rotation deformity of the lumbar vertebrae has been established the psoas muscle on the concave side is acting at a mechanical advantage and will tend to increase the deformity.

The trapezius, rhomboids and lattissimus dorsi all tend to rotate the vertebrae to the opposite side. If again a rotation deformity has been established the muscles on the concave side will be at a mechanical advantage and will tend to increase this.

Synovial joints
Synovial joints are generally categorized according to the shape of their articular surfaces, for example:

(1) Plain joints.
(2) Ball-and-socket joints.
(3) Saddle joints.

In order to design prosthetic joints one must analyse the mechanical functions which the joint serves. Shown in Fig. 3.10 are the three forces and couples which can be applied at a joint. These forces do not act in isolation but generally as a combination which induces sliding and shear movements. To counter these forces, muscles and their tendons that span the joint develop tensile stresses. The design of a joint has to consider the various muscles that act on the joint even if these muscles extend far from the joint.

The application of a force in the anteroposterior or medio-lateral directions or from internal/external rotation couple applied to a joint (Fig 3.10) produces relative sliding of the joint surfaces. Sliding movements are resisted by the soft tissue of the joint.

The magnitude of pressure at the articular surfaces varies directly with the compressive force acting on the joint but varies inversely with the area of contact over which the force is applied. It is important

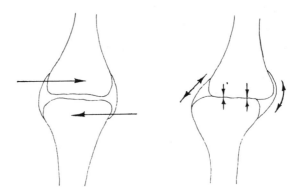

Fig. 3.10 — Three forces and couples applied to a joint producing sliding and wear.

that in designing joints that the contact areas are large enough to transmit the expected loads at pressures which the materials of the joint can withstand. The implant should only transmit compressive stresses across the bone/implant interface. If shear is expected to be transmitted then the implant should be attached to the diaphysis. The bone structure of the diaphysis is designed to resist shear and tension as well as compression stress.

Joint surfaces are very precisely matched in order to transmit loads at the lowest and most uniform pressure. If the articular surface is damaged or removed there is a high probability that osteoarthritis will develop.

Joint stability is maintained by surrounding soft tissue and ligaments. Ligaments are structures in which the tensile force is directly related to their length. In muscle the tensile force can vary independently of their length. The greater the tension in the soft tissue the greater the stability.

FRACTURE HEALING

Natural healing
Consider a simple unsplinted rib fracture. The process of healing can be conveniently divided into three phases: a cellular phase is followed by a phase in which mineralization occurs, and finally the mineralized tissue is exchanged for bone which then remodels.

Cellular phase
Unless movement between fracture fragments can be prevented to a sufficient degree, it is not possible to fill at a single event a fracture gap with a stiff mineralized tissue bound to each fragment. Significant

interfragmentary motion would rupture the mineralized tissue within the fracture gap. Accumulation of a dense mass of cellular callus around the fracture has the effect of sufficiently reducing fracture motion so as to allow mineralization to occur. The stabilizing effect of the cellular callus is primarily dependent on the second moment of area of the callus, or more simply, on the fourth power of its radius. Once the cellular callus achieves a certain degree of stability mineralization can take place. It is a commonplace observation that the more unstable the mechanical environment of a fracture, the greater is the quantity of callus. If the cellular callus is unable to achieve stability in the fracture plane, a non-union of the hypertrophic kind occurs. It can be successfully treated by the imposition of further stability by surgical means, when the non-union plane will be seen to mineralize without the elaboration of any new tissue.

Mineralized phase

Wherever in the callus sufficient conditions of mechanical stability pertain, there mineralization takes place. This determines the typical x-ray appearance of callus which is first visible away from the fracture line and close to the cortical surface. As the cellular callus increases in radius, so the region of sufficient stability approaches the fracture plane. Once callus becomes mineralized, it can be exchanged for woven bone. In those parts which are well supplied with blood, and where mechanical conditions permit, new woven bone is formed in osteoid directly. Where oxygen supply is poor, and mechanical conditions are unstable, the cellular callus will differentiate as cartilage which is later mineralized and exchanged for woven bone. The mineralization of the callus dramatically increases its stiffness, renders obsolete the necessity for its large radius, and allows involution of redundant cellular tissue.

Remodelling phase

Once the fracture fragments have been joined by mineralized tissue with its markedly increased stiffness, woven bone and mineralized cartilage can be exchanged for new lamellar bone which is much more efficient and less bulky for a given amount of strength.

Internal fixation

If the fracture is stabilized adequately using internal plates, no external callus is formed since none is needed and the stimulus of movement is absent, and the fracture heals by the gradual formation of woven bone in the fracture micro-gap. Anatomical reduction is essential so as to avoid fatigue fracture of the implant.

ORTHOTICS

A definition may be derived from the Greek meaning 'in addition' or replacement of a missing part. Orthotics may be from a combination of prosthesis and orthopaedics.

With all orthoses there is a biological response; first the skin where pressure damages the epidermis and dermis, with damage of the circulation if extreme, especially if diabetes, rheumatoid arthritis or any condition that causes a vasculitis is present. The worst end result is ulceration and gangrene.

Heat retention can be a problem with excesss sweating and skin maceration.

There are physical variations amongst individuals and it is not possible to fit everyone into the classical ectomorph, mesomorph, endomorph classification.

Age variations are important, especially in the developing skeleton. The natural history of many conditions is of resolution, e.g. genu valgum, infantile scoliosis.

The American Academy of Orthopedic Surgeons developed a classification of orthoses. These are:

(1) Functional — biomechanical.
(2) Functional — descriptive.

The most practically useful is (2). It consists of three sections:

(a) functional description of patient impairment,
(b) objectives of treatment,
(c) orthotic recommendations.

These can then be subdivided further:

(a)   (i) skeletal bone and joint,
      (ii) neurological sensory and motor,
      (iii) pain,
      (iv) balance,
       (v) skin state,
      (vi) gait deviations,
     (vii) other pathology
(b)   (i) prevention or correction of deformity,
      (ii) reduction of axial load,
      (iii) protection of joints,
      (iv) improvement of ambulation,
       (v) treatment of fractures,
      (vi) other.

(c) The extent of the orthosis is described by the joints over which the orthosis passes. Accordingly, the body is divided into three segments.

Upper limb
S = shoulder
E = elbow
W = wrist
H = hand

Lower limb
H = hip
K = knee
A = ankle
F = foot

Spine
C = cervical
T = thoracic
L = lumbar
SI = sacroiliac

For the hand and foot the symbols MP, PIP, DIP are added and for the thumb CM, MP and IP.

The United Nations usage in combination is adopted, e.g. AFO.

The following symbols are used for designation of control over the function of joints or articulations.

F = free movement
A = assist — application of external force to increase range, velocity or force
R = resist — application of external force to decrease velocity, range or force
S = stop — undesired motion in one direction avoided by a static unit, and when used alone it means restraint of gross movement in neutral position of a joint
V = variable — an adjustable unit not requiring structural change, commonly used with 'stop'
H = hold — elimination of all movement in one plane
L = lock — which is optimal.

All this information is supplied on standard forms.
The desired features of an orthosis should be that it is:

— lightweight,
— reliable,
— good factory manufacture quality control,
— rapidly made and repaired,
— easily adjusted in the clinic,
— hygienic,
— safe from failure and consequent injury to patient,
— accceptable to patient cosmetically,
— acceptable to patient — comfort,
                                        toilet purpose,
                                        ease of application and removal,
                                        low energy use,
                                        not damaging to clothes.

Regional orthoses
Cervical spine — conditions that require an orthosis:

— cervical spondylosis,
— rheumatoid arthritis,
— infection,
— trauma,
— osteoporosis,
— neoplastic, primary and secondary
— neurological weakness,
— vertebro-basilar insufficiency.

The aims of treatment are to:

— reduce inflammation and spasm,
— reduce compressive stress,
— stabilize joints,
— limit joint movement range,
— reduce heat loss

There are many types of orthosis varying from collars which pass around the neck alone, to braces extending from pelvis or chest to skull. The plastic foam collar is easily available but has poor control of movement whereas the plastic rigid collar has better control of movement.

Occasionally a brace plus a headband is required for high collapsing disease of the upper cervical spine.

Thoracic spine

If the centre of mass of the whole body can be calculated and if the mobile articulation is known, the degree of correction to produce stability can be determined.

Lumbar spine

Lumbar orthoses make up 30% of the total number of orthotic prescriptions in the UK per annum and 25% of the total budget.

There are over fifty different types of variable function but usually they seem to function as a placebo. Biomechanically, it is thought that incorporation of a small band around the pelvis has its greatest effect by:

(1) Diminishing the posterior subluxation of the facet joints.
(2) To promote beneficial posture.
(3) To limit the wedge-like action of the sacrum in relationship to the sacroiliac joints under the effect of body weight.

These effects give clinical credence to the narrow leather belt around the pelvis of manual workers earlier this century and modern day weight-lifters. In both cases, they are designed to limit back pain.

Scoliosis

The mechanical problems are that there are multiple small deformed segments, making it difficult to concentrate a correcting force. Also, the site of application of a correcting force is a long way from the site of deformity.

In addition, the deformity requires correction in all planes, while variable pathologies acting on the growing skeleton make for forces that are difficult to correct.

Plaster of paris was initially used to correct the deformity but because of the forces generated was discontinued in favour of the Milwaukee brace and its more modern Boston brace. The advent of modern materials have helped enormously in their evolution.

Hand and wrist orthoses are commonly used for trauma, rheumatoid arthritis and neurological conditions. The problems, however, are:

— swelling,
— stiffness,
— finger position related to ligament laxity (need to immobilize with ligaments in a tense position),
— maintaining the transverse arches of the hand.

The function of these orthoses are to:

— provide dynamic splintage to exercise muscles and joints,
— correct fixed deformities,
— rest in a particular position.

Shoulder orthoses

The indications for these are pain, trauma and neurological flaccid paralysis. The aims of treatment are to relieve pain and to stabilize the shoulder and elbow which may be flaccid after brachial plexus injuries. The two most commonly used braces are the Roehampton flail arm splint and the Rancho-Log Amigos hospital brachial plexus brace.

Hip orthoses

Congential dislocation of the hip is treated using either a von Rosen's splint or a Pavlick harness (Fig. 3.11). In Perthes' disease the aim is

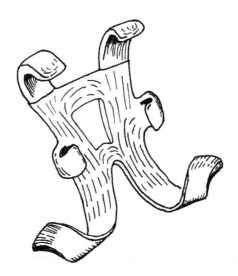

Fig. 3.11 — Von Rosen splint used in the treatment of congenital dislocation of the hip during the first two months of life.

the relief of compressive stress which is achieved by by-passing the hip through a crutch. Several are used, the most common being the Snyder sling, Birmingham splint, Toronto Perthes' orthosis and the Scotish-Rite Perthes' orthosis.

The foot

Flat foot is a common condition which is frequently self-correcting. However, the hypermobile hyperproviated type needs to be treated actively with an outside iron and inside Y strap to school age and then an extended heel cup or Rose–Schwarts meniscus.

Spasmodic valgus can have a sudden onset in early adolescence, boys are more affected than girls, possibly related to a calcaneo-navicular impingement or bar. The foot is in maximum pronation and tight achilles. The treatment involves the removal of the bar before twelve years of age and stretch the tendoachilles and maintain the position with an outside iron and inside Y strap or an extended heel cup. Treatment must continue for several years to get good results.

Rheumatoid arthritis causes pronation of the foot which if it remains correctable can be treated with an inside iron and T strap.

Cavus feet are reasonably common of which there are two main types:

(1) The high arched pronated foot which is treated with an outside iron and Y strap or an extended heel cup.
(2) The progressive cavus which is a neurogenic foot with clawing of toes, inversion and sometimes vascular and sensory deficiencies which predispose to ulceration. This condition is treated with a multilayer thermoplastic insole for relief of pressure and a rigid sole for relief of shear. An orthopaedic boot must be prescribed for severe degrees of cavus. If one has a narrow heel, then increased stability can be obtained with a floated out heel. Due to the turning moment about the subtalar joint and ankle joint during supination and the inability of os calcis to roll outwards, great forces are applied to the shoe. In these cases, a short medial iron and lateral Y strap are recommended.

Painful heel syndrome

A Rose–Parker insole rolls the os calcis inwards without applying pressure to the tender area, as the plantar fascia is closely applied to the periosteum to join with the achilles tendon.

Metatarsalgia

Two types of this condition are common:

(1) Maldistribution of weight sharing under the metatarsal heads.
(2) Morton's metatarsalgia.

Both these conditions can be relieved by an insole carrying a metatarsal dome behind the callosity or pain. However, an increasingly larger size will be necessary as skin and tissue atrophy. If the toes are squeezed against the uppers then a three-quarter sole may be tried. The severe cases may require a metatarsal bar (Fig. 3.12).

Below knee orthoses

These are commonly prescribed and the main types are of metal and leather, plastic, or a combination of both materials. Their main functions are:

(1) To limit movement range.
(2) To stabilize the foot.
(3) To exert a knee control function.
(4) To relieve longitudinal or lateral forces.

Long leg orthoses

These are used for partial or total relief of weight from the hip. Also, to relieve stress within the leg in a longitudinal, lateral and torsional direction. Also, stabilization of the knee in a sagittal and coronal plane, in addition, to complete or partial limitation of movement within the knee and exerting hip control function.

Modern design and the use of plastic materials has significant advantages. These include approximately 50% saving in weight, improved hygiene and some improved cosmesis.

(Cast brace) or functional brace

The general guidelines are that this brace should be painless on minor movements, with no shortening or longitudinal compression; that angulation produced by forces is elastic and self-correcting with longitudinal shortening not exceeding a half-inch for the femur and a quarter-inch for the tibia.

Holding the fracture position is dependent upon the three-point fixation and soft tissue hinge with hydrodynamic total contact containment.

Knee orthoses

These are usually prescribed for:

(1) The elderly with rheumatoid or osteoarthritis.
(2) The young with ligamentous instability.

The mechanical problems are:

(1) Short lever arms.
(2) The point of application of resisting forces is frequently over soft tissue.
(3) Maintaining correct vertical and rotational position.

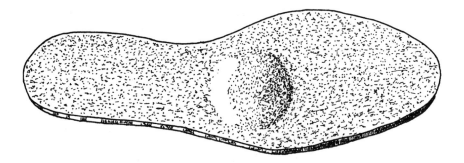

Fig. 3.12 — Insole for shoe with metatarsal dome to take weight behind the
metatarsal heads.

(4) To secure a fixed point of reaction to a theoretical action in
    rotation.

   The aims of treatment are:

(1) Rest in a position as near to full extension as possible.
(2) Stabilization of the knee.
(3) Control of joint range.
(4) Comfort and freedom from compression.

Stabilization of the knee

There are two different types of knee instability:

(1) Ligamentous laxity.
(2) Change of joint axis by bone collapse or loss of articular cartilage
    or meniscus.

   With ligamentous laxity you must assess whether the knee is
intrinsically stable enough to be stabilized. With joint axis change you
must overcome axis alignment and control valgus and varus
deformity.
   To resist longitudinal rotation on knee flexion a very robust
device is needed. It is used post-operatively and in American football
and skiing.

Combined trunk and body brace

(1) Poliomyelitis causing widespread flaccid paralysis without sen-
    sory loss.
(2) Spastic and athetoid cerebral palsy.
(3) Traumatic or congenital paraplegic conditions.

   The functional requirements are:

(1) Intrinsic and extrinsic stabilization of the skeleton.
(2) Control of hip joint movement during walking.

Types of combined trunk and body brace:

(1) The swivel walker.
(2) Hip guidance orthosis.
(3) Reciprocating gait orthosis which uses cables or gearbox to attempt to transfer energy from one leg to another.

These are all highly specialized orthoses and their prescription should only be undertaken by a specialist with much experience in their particular subject.

GAIT

Walking has two phases, swing and stance, occurring simultaneously in opposite legs and sequentially in the same leg. There are two phases of double stance each 13% of total cycle, starting at the commencement of toe and heel rocker of each leg.

Running starts when there are no double-stance phases.

Stride length is ground covered between beginning and end of one completed phase of one leg.

Step length is the distance one foot moves in front of the other.

Components of gait

(1) Pendulum action — flexion-extension action of the swing leg.
(2) Vaulting action of stance leg.
(3) Pelvic movements — horizontal rotation
                                       vertical rotation
                                       lateral movement.
(4) Knee — there are two phases of flexion during the gait cycle:
     (a) heel contact — shock absorption,
     (b) prior to toe off and during swing gait concerned with the clearance of the swing leg.
(5) Foot–ankle complex — the three rockers occur in succession with some overlap:
     (a) heel rocker,
     (b) ankle rocker,
     (c) toe rocker.

Plantar fascia mechanism is shortened and tightened each time phalangeal extension occurs. This is usually twice in each gait cycle.

Anatomically, it has its origin at the calcaneum posteriorly and five slips anteriorly inserted into the base of the proximal phalanx.

Active extension of toes at heel strike — this causes the medial arch to rise the most and consequently supination of the foot. Muscle controlled de-extension of the toes occurs as the foot reaches the ground. This provides some shock absorption function.

Toe rocker then converts the foot into a rigid structure by repeating the previous action passively and thereby playing a part in the control of rise and fall of the body centre of mass. The shape of the foot is not constant and this must be taken into account in orthotic design.

FRACTURE MANAGEMENT

The management of fractures depends upon reduction and immobilization.

Reduction

Closed technique by which the mechanism of injury is reversed; therefore, an understanding of the mechanism of injury is vital.

Open technique is a preliminary to operative fixation.

Immobilization — extracorporeal

Plaster of paris: holds fracture to length, prevents varus and valgus deformity, and prevents rotatory movements if the joints above and below are immobilized.

The advantages are that it is cheap. The disadvantages are that it is weak, cracks easily, and is not waterproof. Therefore, modern materials based on fibreglass or thermoplastics are used but they are expensive.

Cast bracing:

(1) The fracture must be painless on minor movements.
(2) No shortening or longitudinal compression.
(3) Angulation produced by forces is elastic and self-correcting.
(4) Shortening should not exceed a half-inch for femur or a quarter-inch for tibia.

Traction: the aim is to apply a force sufficient to overcome the spasm in the muscle around the fractured bone. This disimpacts the bone ends, diminishes the crepitus and consequently pain. The force is applied either via the skin as skin traction but it is not as efficient as skeletal traction which is applied via a pin directly through a bone in the affected limbs but not the fractured bone because of the danger of sepsis.

To each action there must be an opposite reaction to balance the forces. This can sometimes be body weight or the reaction of a splint against a bony interface.

External fixation

These are called frames and are designed to hold the fractured fragments rigidly and in anatomical alignment until the repair and healing of the soft tissue is complete.

Frames can be:

(1) *Unilateral*. These do not provide absolute rigidity during weight bearing because the varus force on the tibia does cause some angulatory movement. They, therefore, neutralize only rotatory and axial loading.
(2) *Bilateral*. These are more rigid and neutralize rotatary axial and varus valgus forces but not all anteroposterior forces.
(3) *A frame*. This is a very rigid structure and neutralizes movement in all planes.

Internal fixation

Rigid plates

These aim to restore exact anatomical continuity and allow primary bone healing. The principle is the exact reconstruction of the tube of bone using small interfragmentary lag screws (Fig. 3.13) and then using the plate as a neutralizer of the forces across the fracture site.

If the opposite side of the bone to the plate is not perfectly constituted then the bone will bend under the forces of weight bearing or movement. This cyclical loading will be taken by the plate which will eventually fracture. (Refer to Chapter 1, Cyclical fatigue.) This may occur at any time up to 18 months.

Flexible plates

To overcome this problem, plates with some degree of flexibility have been developed. Modern materials and technology have resulted in the carbon plate with alternate layers of carbon and epoxy resin. They allow several degrees of movement and consequently enable rapid bone union by external callus on the opposite side to the plate initially.

Intra-medullary nails

This technique allows the fracture to be splinted longitudinally thus neutralizing varus and valgus but allowing some axial compression (Fig. 3.14). When the fracture is not in the middle third of the bone, it allows rotation. The problem with comminuted fractures is that axial

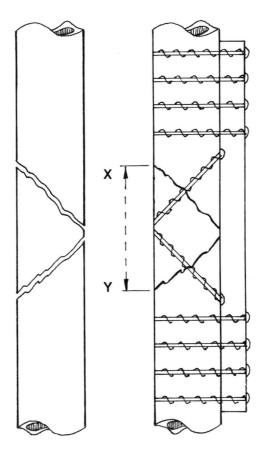

Fig. 3.13 — Illustrates a fracture of a long bone, the two components of which are held with two interfragmentary lag screws and a metal plate on the outside of the bone neutralizing the forces across the fracture.

compression will cause shortening of the bone. The interlocking nail has been designed to neutralize the axial and rotatory forces when the fracture is in the upper or lower third (Fig. 3.15).

PROSTHESES

Total hip replacement

Femoral side

The femoral shaft must be reamed to a size adequate to accept the prosthesis. Blood is removed. Then it is irrigated with saline, preferably under pressure using a brush which can be inserted down the femoral shaft. It is then irrigated with hydrogen peroxide to help

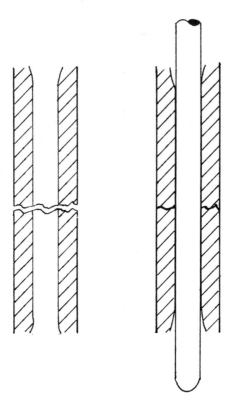

Fig. 3.14 — Transverse fracture of middle third of long bone, also splinted with
intramedullary nail showing grip above and below fracture site.

reduce bleeding and protect against anaerobic organisms. A bone or
plastic cement plug is inserted into the femoral shaft 2 cm further,
then the tip of the prosthesis. The cement is then introduced using a
cement gun starting distally and working proximally. This ensures
that the cement is introduced evenly and that no blood is mixed with
the cement to produce lamellation and reduce the strength (Fig.
3.16).

The space between the femoral shaft and the prosthesis must be
completely filled with no areas of lamellation from blood or air or
bone fragments otherwise these will cause stress concentrations.

Acetabular side

Here the bone is prepared to reveal raw cancellous bone. All bone
fragments and blood must be removed, then the bone cement can key
into the bone. The keying can cause cement penetration up to 2 mm
into the bone. This helps the acetabulum and bone cement to resist
deforming forces.

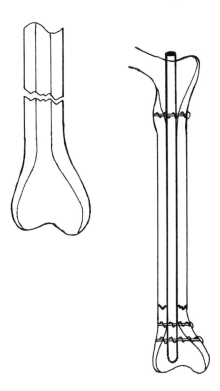

Fig. 3.15 — The locking screws at both ends of the nail are used to prevent rotation of
the bone around the nail where the diameter of the medulla is greater than the nail.

The knee

The same criteria apply to the femoral and tibial surfaces. As a
tourniquet is used, blood is not involved, but fat and bone fragments
are. Fat is removed with fat emulsifiers, e.g. Savlon saline. These
techniques leave a very clean cancellous bone surface for keying and
to resist the forces.

Materials of hip and bone prostheses

The aims must be:

(1) Low coefficient of friction.
(2) High resistance to wear.
(3) Strong enough to resist deforming forces.

The coefficient of friction is related to the nature of the surfaces in
contact and their surface areas. The smaller the surface area in
contact, the lower the friction. In the hip this is practically achieved
by decreasing the size of the femoral head to as small as is practically
possible (Fig. 3.17).

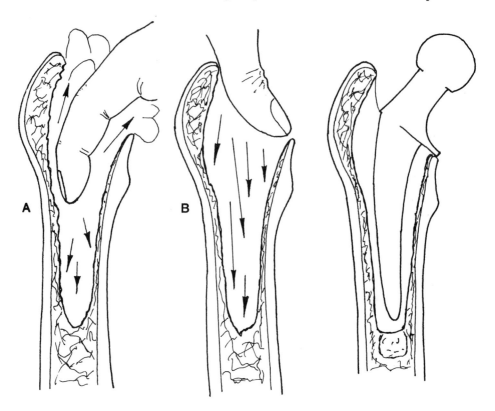

Fig. 3.16 — Showing cement inserted by finger pushing A+B and the inserted
prosthesis with cement plug.

Initial prostheses were metal on metal but these suffered loosening due to high frictional resistance. To overcome this, one of the
components is now made of high density polyethylene. This lowers
friction — wear is very slight. In the hip, if one walks the average of
four million walk cycles per year, then the acetabular wear is 0.1 mm
per year.

Bone–cement interface
The keying of cement into the bone is vital, therefore the two points
of weakness are the bone–cement and the cement–prosthesis inter-
faces, and any defect in the cement caused by faulty cementing
technique. Figure 3.18 shows the deforming forces upon these areas.

Positioning of the prosthesis is vital. If they are not correctly
orientated then the forces can be increased and failure of the
prosthesis occurs more rapidly.

The evaluation of joint replacement was due to a better under-

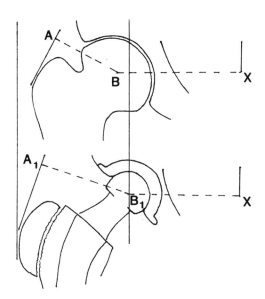

Fig. 3.17 — Shows large head size 28 mm (B) and small head size 22 mm(B_1) and
their respective distances from the centre of gravity of the body (BX and B_1 X) and
the length of the abductor lever arm (AB and A_1B_1).

standing of biomechanics. Early prostheses squeaked due to the
increased friction between the acrylic and the acetabulum. Joint
replacement has become successful because of:

(1) Stable weight-bearing surfaces.
(2) Low friction between components.
(3) Secure fix to bone with bone cement.
(4) The surgeon knowing the biomechanical principles with, in
    addition, a knowledge of materials and design.

The components of joint replacement must survive cyclical loading up to 3–5 times body weight in order to avoid the main causes of
failure which are:

(1) Infection.
(2) Dislocation.
(3) Loosening of the femoral or acetabular components.
(4) Failure of the femoral stem.

The surgeon must:

(1) Perform the procedure correctly.

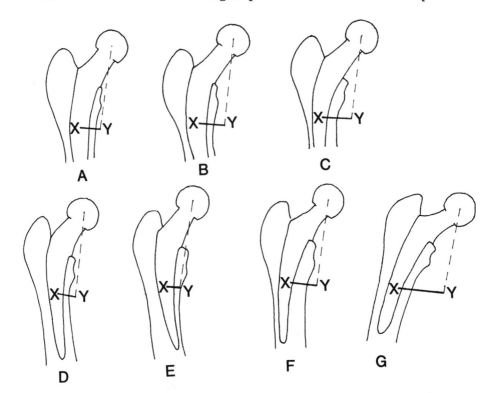

Fig. 3.18 — Shows the deforming moment arm (XY) in the correct position (B) and
with too much varus (G) or too much valgus (E).

(2) Manage problems.
(3) Select components intelligently.
(4) Counsel patients concerning their physical activities.

The forces acting on the hip

Since the length of the body weight lever arm to abductors is 2.5:1,
you need 2.5 times the body weight pull in the abductors to keep the
pelvis level while standing on one leg.

Three times the body weight on the femoral head during the
stance phase of gait, i.e. sum of forces in abductors plus body weight.
(When running it may be times 10.)

Therefore, body weight increase or physical weight increase add
to forces that loosen, bend or break the femoral component.

The forces act not only in the coronal plane but rotate and bend
the femoral stem posteriorly (because the centre of rotation is
posterior to the axis of the joint). These latter two forces increase
when the hip is flexed, e.g. getting up from a chair, climbing stairs or
incline, or lifting (Fig. 3.19).

The abductor lever arm is shortened in arthritis of the hip joint where the ratio of body weight to abductors is 4:1. But in the antalgic gait the centre of gravity is moved laterally to the affected hip and thus decreases the body weight lever arm, making the abductors' body weight ratio 1:1.

Varus and valgus position

The valgus position (more than 140°) decreases the bending moment but proportionally increases the axial loading of the stem. This is a desirable position but shortens the abductor lever arm. However, when the valgus is excessive, it may increase the strain on knee and ankle.

Varus position increases the bending moment and decreases the axial loading on the stem. Also, it lengthens the abductor lever arm, but must be avoided as it increases loosening and stem failure. It also shortens the femur and can result in dislocation.

A moderate valgus is generally better than varus but ideally the femoral neck shaft angle should be 140°.

Cross-section, curve and stem length

The prosthesis must resist tensile and rotatory forces. The middle third of the prosthesis resists the majority of the tensile forces.

The area of contact between cement and prosthesis must be increased maximally without sharp edges as these cause an increase in high stress concentration and cause cement fracture.

Maximum tensile strength

The prosthetic stem will break at this point and is determined by:

(1) Stem design.
(2) Direction of the load applied.
(3) Varus and valgus orientation of stem in canal.
(4) The level at which stem is held firmly.

If the stem is firmly cemented into the canal then the area of maximum stress is best if on the prosthesis surface. If the area of maximum stress is within the cement, then this can fracture as it is subjected to a higher tensile strength than it can withstand in this mode.

If the proximal third of the stem is not securely fixed, then the prosthesis will fracture just proximal to the area of firm fix.

If only the distal third is fixed, then the stem fails at a more distal level.

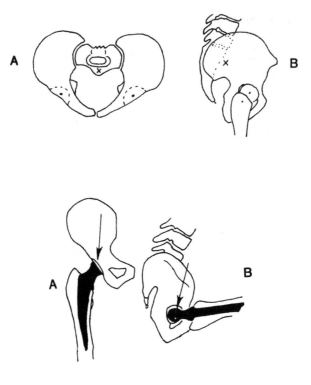

Fig. 3.19 — Shows relevant position of centre of gravity behind hip joint axis and the forces on femoral component during full flexion of hip joint.

Femoral head diameter

The load per unit area is greater with a small femoral head (i.e. 22 mm); the frictional resistance is less.

Coefficient of friction and frictional torque

The coefficient of friction is a measure of resistance in moving one object over another; it varies with materials used, the finish of the surfaces, the temperature, and whether tested dry or with lubricant. The coefficient of friction in normal joints is 0.008 to 0.02. Metal in contact with high density polyethylene is 0.02 which is very close to normal.

Frictional torque

This is when the loaded joint is passed through an arc of motion. The frictional torque is transferred to the cup, stem, cement bone interface as a force that tends to twist the components. The frictional torque may crack or move the whole cement mass. Therefore, any movement of cement or increase of shear force at the cement–bone interface causes bone absorption. This shows the theoretical advantage of a small femoral head over a large one.

Wear
The determining factors are:

(1) Coefficient of friction and finish of surfaces.
(2) Boundary lubrication.
(3) Load or pressure.
(4) Distance travelled each cycle.
(5) Number of cycles

The wear rate is unaffected by pressure of approximately $50 \, kg/cm^2$ or less. It is directly proportional to abrasion rather than adhesive or corrosive factors.
The important factors appear to be:

(1) The number of cycles.
(2) Any surface wear.
(3) The material (the metal femoral head sustains minimal wear but the high density polyethylene in the acetabulum wears at approximately 0.07 mm/year).

Lubrication
This is by boundary lubrication whereby the boundary lubricant decreases friction by interacting with the surfaces (i.e. synovial fluid).

Materials
Femoral stem failure is caused by:

(1) Weight and activity of patient.
(2) Loss of support of cement in bone.
(3) Poor design and position of component.
(4) Wrong type of metal used.

The most important reference terms are the:

(1) Yield strength.
(2) Fatigue strength.
(3) Ultimate tensile strength.
(4) Corrosion.

Stainless steel is more ductile than other alloys and the most common cause of a fractured stem is repeated loadings less than the yield strength but more than the fatigue limit which produces an incomplete fracture that may progress to a fracture.

Ideal femoral implant
The above must have:

(1) High fatigue limit.
(2) High yield strength.
(3) Ultimate tensile strength.
(4) Young's modulus, if:
    (a) low you get more frequent bone and cement failure,
    (b) high you get more disine osteoporosis with loosening of the stem.
(5) Biocompatibility:
    (a) it must be non-allergenic from chrome, cobalt or nickel,
    (b) no sterile inflammation that may cause loosening,
    (c) no systemic carcinogenic effects.
(6) Corrosion — in the saline environment of the body there is more resistance in polished than unpolished surfaces. Stainless steel corrodes more easily than cobalt or titanium alloys in a given electrolyte. Chrome and molybdenum produce a corrosion resistant surface layer to stainless steel. All metallic implants are passivated using nitric acid to form an oxide on their surface to resist corrosion.

Metal characteristics
(1) Stainless steel with low impurities and passivated finish is entirely suitable for implantation.
(2) Cobalt-based alloys are highly resistant to corrosion; galvanic corrosion occurs but less than in stainless steel. They may be resistant to fatigue and cracking from corrosion, but may suddenly fail because of brittleness.
(3) Titanium and titanium based alloys have excellent resistance to corrosion, fatigue and failure. The titanium alloys contain vanadium or aluminium. Therefore, you must be wary of Alzheimer's disease with the latter.

Acetabulum component

This is made from ultra-high molecular weight polyethylene which is viscoelastic and exhibits creep or deformation under loads which is minimized by containing the cup within rigid boundaries, e.g. the acetabular cavity or metal backing with regard to the knees.

The acetabulum component can be manufactured by machining and compression moulding. The sterilizing technique can only be gamma-radiation as autoclaving causes permanent softening and deformation and ethylene oxide does not permeate the interior of the material.

Clinical experience shows it to be well tolerated after fifteen years and produces a thin fibrous capsule, no inflammatory reaction and no evidence of carcinogenesis.

Polymethyl methacrylate (bone cement)

Polymethyl methacrylate (PMMA) is a cold or self-curing acrylic polymer. It is the weakest link in the bone cement/implant composite, and has known chemical and physical properties. Curing occurs when the powder which contains a catalyst is added to the liquid which contains an accelerator.

Its function is to fix components to bone and transfer forces to larger surfaces, therefore, decreasing the pressure per unit area.

It does not bond to polished surfaces but does to cancellous surfaces especially when forced into the interstices when soft. A secure bond is important as movement at the cement–bone interface causes absorption of bone and loosening of cement.

The PMMA can withstand considerable compression forces but fails under tension or shear forces. It is three times stronger under compression than tension and is half the strength of compact bone.

Shear and tension forces are produced if bone is resorbed because of motion, infection or any other cause such as insufficient support due to osteoporosis or rheumatoid arthritis.

Tissue effects of PMMA

(1) The temperature of polymerization is 67°C.
(2) Occlusion of the nutrient metaphyseal arteries may produce bone necrosis.
(3) Cytotoxic and lipolytic effects of non-polymerized monomer.

The temperature of the exothermic reaction at the bone-cement interface can be as high as 70°C, some is dissipated by the prosthesis and some by the local circulation.

Cement technique

The principle is preparation of the bone surface to allow keying of the cement into the cancellous surface.

Time scale

(1) 0–3 weeks — up to 3 mm thick tissue damage.
(2) 3 weeks–2 years — ingrowth of fibrous tissue and capillaries that replaces necrotic bone.
(3) 2 years onward — the bed is well established at 0.5–1.5 mm thick space containing round fragments of PMMA with giant-cell response. Larger masses of PMMA set more slowly and are 80% strong after 15 minutes with maximal final strength after 18 hours.

A cement plug is essential to have a firm column of cement for maximal strength, with no blood or air in the shaft of bone. A 4 mm thick column around the entire femoral stem is essential to:

(1) Distribute load to as large a surface area as possible.
(2) To make the cement thick enough to resist fragmentation.

A continuous cuff of cement firmly packed between medial surface of prosthesis and proximal femur. If little or no cement is securely trapped between bone and prosthesis then the following may occur:

(1) Bone absorption.
(2) Cement fragmentation.
(3) Stem failure.

The medial cement must rest on cancellous bone or cortical bone and *not* on marrow or loose cancellous bone (Fig. 3.20).
The cement must extend 1–2 cm distal to the tip of the stem as this is where the stem is subject to axial loading.

Alternatives to PMMA

(1) Proplast — polytetrafluoroethylene.
(2) Porous polyethylene.
(3) Ceramics — low friction, good wear but brittle, tensile characteristics poor.

Material selection
Plastics:

(1) Lightweight.
(2) Mouldability.
(3) Resistance to chemical attack.
(4) Ease of fabrication and moulding.
(5) Cosmetic.

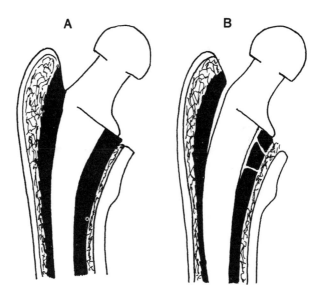

Fig. 3.20 — Shows normal cement column under femoral component and the crumbling of the cement that occurs if it is placed on cancellous bone on the calcar.

Metals:
(1) High strength.
(2) High stiffness.
(3) Stable characteristics at ambient temperatures.
(4) High energy absorption before failure.

FURTHER READING

Backman, S., The proximal end of the femur, *Acta Radial.*, **146**, 1–166, 1957.

Markoff, K. L., Deformation of the thoracolumbar intevertebral joints in response to external loads — a biomechanical study using autopsy material, *J. Bone Joint Surg.*, **54A**, 511–533, 1972.

Nicoll, E. A., Fractures of the dorsolumbar spine, *J. Bone Joint Surg.*, **31B**, 376–394, 1949.

Pennal, G., Stress studies of the lumbar spine, *J. Bone Joint Surg.*, **48B**, 18, 1966.

Rockwood, C. A. and Green D. P., *Fractures*, Vol. 2, J. B. Lippincott Company, Toronto, 1975.

Weil, G. C., Price, E. M. and Rusbridge, H. W., The diagnosis and treatment of fractures of the pelvis and their complications, *Amer. J. Surg.*, **44**, 108–116, 1939.

Glossary

Presented here are a few medical terms which the engineer may not be familiar with.

Abduct   To draw away from the middle line of the body.

Alzheimer's disease   Form of presenile dementia.

Annulus fibrosis   Peripheral part of intervertebral disc.

Anterior   Front of body or limb.

Avulsion   The forcible separation of two parts.

Biocompatibility   Ease in which foreign substance can be placed in the human body without adverse effects.

Bronchial plexus   Nerves belonging to the upper arm.

Comminution   Fracture of a bone into a number of pieces.

Coronal plane   A vertical plane at right angles to the medial plane.

Differentiation   The acquisition of a distinct or separate character.

Dorsal   Related to the back of an organ or body.

Dura   Outermost membrane which lines the interior of the skull.

Ectomorph/mesomorph/endomorph   Types of build of the human body.

Flexion   To bend.

Foramina   Hole or aperture.

Hypertrophy   Increase in size.

Interstices   Small spaces or crevices present between parts of the body.

Kyphosis   Outward curvature of the spine causing hunching of the back.

Lordosis   Inward curvature of the spine.

Median plane   Anteroposterior plane dividing body into two halves.

Meniscus   Semilunar cartilage of the knee.

Metaphyseal   Part of long bone between shaft and end.

Osteoporosis   Bone disease that results in reduced quantity of bone.

Posterior   Back of body or limb.

Sternum   Bone in anterior midline of rib cage.

Subluxation   Incomplete dislocation.

Sagittal plane   An anteroposterior plane.

Ventral   Towards the front.

Varus   Legs are bent outwards.

Valgus   Displacement outwards from the central line of the body.

Tendoachilles   Connective tissue with which the calf muscle attaches to the heel.

Index